The book deals with the causes, cure & prevention of certain Hair maladies such as Dandruff & Itchy scalps, Hair-loss/Baldness, untimely greying of Hair, Lice problem, Boils & Split-end Hair etc. and also lay emphasis, in particular, on their treatment by Yogasanas & Acupressure.

It enlightens us about Hair-Care basics & products, Home-made solutions, Hairstyles, Clever Cutting Techniques, Perming, Dyeing & Colouring, Cleansing & Conditioning of Hair.

The book provides useful informations on diet for keeping hair healthy.

Hair Care

[Prevention of Dandruff & Baldness]

Dr. Renu Gupta

Diamond Pocket Books

ISBN : 81-7182-122-7

© Publisher

Publisher	:	**Diamond Pocket Books (P) Ltd.**
		X-30, Okhla Industrial Area, Phase-II
		New Delhi-110020
Phone	:	011-41611861
Fax	:	011-41611866
E-mail	:	sales@diamondpublication.com
Website	:	www.diamondpublication.com
Edition	:	2006
Price	:	75.00
Printer	:	Aadarsh Printers,
		Navin Shahdara, Delhi- 32

Hair-Care   **Rs. 75/-**

By : Dr. Renu Gupta

Preface

Traditionally it used to be the female folk that evinced more care for its hair but that age is now long past. In a world that is becoming increasingly 'gender-free' at least in appearances with famous male celebrities sporting ponytails and renowned actresses preferring 'crew-cuts'—any book on hair-care is not supposed to cater only one gender group. Hence this book is unique in the sense that it tries to analyse and offer solutions to also basically male hair problems like dandruff, thinning and hair-loss. An attempt has also been made to offer scientific causes and physio-psychological explanations to certain hair maladies.

Various modern 'hair-dos' and ancient 'kesh-vinyas' have also been illustrated with a view to offering a wide choice before our readers. Much emphasis has been placed on 'home-made' solutions to the hair-problems since they have successfully withstood the test of time. Hence, it can be claimed that no dimension of hair-care has been left uncovered in this book. Moreover, hair has been dealt not in exclusivity but as a part of the organic whole of human personality. It is hoped that our discerning readership would give this work a warm welcome. The author is particularly grateful to Mr. Narendra Kumar, Managing Director of Diamond Pocket Books, for providing every freedom and help in the compilation of this book.

Dr. Renu Gupta

Contents

1

Hair : The Crown of the Beautiful : General Care

To many grown ups, bunch of hair is a useless pile one carries on the head. Of course hair is not as necessary to the body as eye-ear-nose or even skin would appear. You don't see with your hair, don't eat with its help and it hardly adds to your perceptive power. On the contrary the lush growth of hair around the ears might disturb your audio perception. But is hair really useless ? Don't curls add to your beauty and charm ? Won't you go a long way to have your hair properly trimmed to add beauty to your face ? Hair does and hence we find literature full of adulatory descriptions of it. To some its bunch might appear like the dark cobras, to other like thick rain-ladden clouds covering a moon-like face. In fact, hair is the most versatile and permanent accessory of a human being, particularly to women. It is a vital part of her looks and her personality. Hair gives a frame to a women's face, complements her life style, accentuates her fashion appeal and charms. To a cosmopolitan being hair is a fluid medium of self-expression and art—a manifestation of own hidden aesthetical preferences.

It is on account of this reason that a person who appreciates good looks and great hair styles also recognises the merit in taking a good care of it. But before we talk more about it let us know what is hair ?

HAIR BASICS

There are hair-care techniques and products that can noticeably improve the appearance of your hair. But you just always remember the following facts about hair :

On average hair grows about 2.5 cm (1 in) per month, with the strongest growth period for women being between the ages of 14 and 40, when you also produce the most oestrogen. But your hair never stops growing, it just slows down as you get older.

A strand of hair is made up of three layers— medulla, cortex and cuticle.

The medulla runs the length of the hair shaft, but is often broken at intervals and sometimes people with fine hair have no medulla at all. Its exact purpose is unknown, though its presence or absence seems to make little difference to what you can do with your hair.

The cortex makes up between 75 and 90 per cent of the hair shaft, containing cells that affect the elasticity and strength of your hair and pigments giving it its colour.

The outer layer, the cuticle, is made of flat, overlapping scales that provide a protective covering for the other layers. When these scales lie flat, light bounces off them easily, making the hair look shiny.

The hairs grow out of follicles in the scalp, at the base of which lie the papillae. These absorb nutrients from the blood supply. As soon as a new hair surfaces from the follicle, through the skin, the cells die and harden (keratinize). All visible hair is then, in effect, dead.

Hair is made of strong elastic strands of proteins called 'Keratin' and in chemical terms is composed of oxygen, iron, nitrogen, hydrogen, sulphur, carbon and phosphorus. The exact proportions of these chemical elements vary with sex, age, type and colour of hair.

The sources of hair are very small tiny pockets in our skin and scalp known as 'follicles'. These follicles are not evenly spread on the scalp but are found together in groups of two to five each. Every follicle follows a life cycle of its own, producing six inches of hair a year, for as long as four years, before it falls out. This starts all over again after a short period.

The basal-tip of the hair in scalp is known as 'Papilla' which is a small out-growth of the skin, shaped like a door-knob and lying at the tip of the follicle. The Papilla contains the blood vessel to supply nourishment to the hair.

During the active period, the new cell growth pushes the older part of the hair away from the Papilla until it falls out. It is the pattern of cell growth at the Papilla which determines whether hair growth would be straight, wavy or curly.

The following diagram would give you a better idea about the structure of hair.

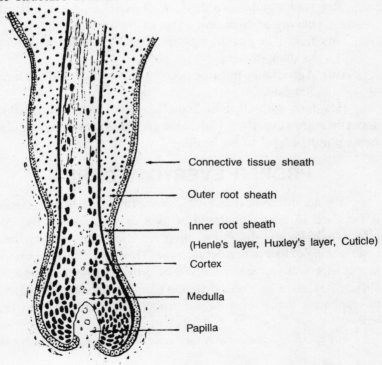

- Connective tissue sheath
- Outer root sheath
- Inner root sheath (Henle's layer, Huxley's layer, Cuticle)
- Cortex
- Medulla
- Papilla

11

The pattern of growth usually becomes uneven during adolescence when the growth of hair peaks only to decline as we grow older. The cell growth pattern can change otherwise due to illness, drugs, pregnancy etc.

WHAT MAKES HAIR LOOK HEALTHY ?

Although many theories have been advanced to define characteristics of a healthy hair growth, you may be surprised that till date no hair-expert, cosmetologist or trichologist has been able to comprehensively and conclusively describe all the characteristics of healthy hair. Nevertheless, some of the most common characteristics, widely believed to be reliable are the following :

(i) Hair should appear thick and dense, fine and silky which means not too oily or rough.

(ii) Hair should give the look of their being lustre-filled, having a shine and gloss of their own.

(iii) It must be pliable, capable of setting and styling suiting to their owner.

(iv) Appearance must be bouncy, full-bodied and not limp and lank.

However, with all these conditions you must feel satisfied about their growth pattern. Unless the growth is proper and regular hair cannot be said to be healthy.

PROPER EVERYDAY CARE

It is not different than taking care of the skin. After all hair is believed to be the extreme of skin bristles essentially. An effective hair-care discipline involves cleansing, toning and conditioning of hair in regular intervals. However, most important aspect of effective care is the use of proper hair-care products. Different types of hair need different hair-care products. Needless to emphasise that use of wrong products is detrimental to the hair.

Foremost routine in daily hair-care is cleansing. The purpose of cleansing is to wash away excess oil on hair and scalp and clear the hair follicles from dead cells. Proper cleansing encourages healthy hair growth.

When you have cleansed your hair, the scalp and hair need the tonic exercise. The toning of scalp and hair is achieved by gently massaging the head. This helps in stimulating and invigorating the blood circulation essential for healthy growth.

What people generally forget is the fact that most important part of hair-care is conditioning. It is actually a part of the restorative routine. If the hair is excessively stripped of moisture or oil due to harsh cleansing, or application of harsh chemicals such as perm lotions etc. The conditioning routine aims at restoring and correcting the imbalance. This kind of condition depends on the physical conditioning of the hair.

CLEANSING AND CONDITIONING TIPS

It is important to get the basics of hair-care–shampooing, conditioning, drying and brushing-right, if you are to avoid problems that will take time to correct later.

Shampoo

Choosing a shampoo that works for you is often a trial-and-error process, but there are some useful guidelines :

- ○ Pick a shampoo that is designed for your hair type as this should leave your hair feeling clean and looking shiny (shampoo should not leave any stickiness behind or dull the hair).
- ○ Never use washing-up liquid or household detergent on your hair as they are highly alkaline and disturb your hair's pH balance.
- ○ Avoid having a common family shampoo—the chances are that everyone will have a different hair type—so buy a selection.
- ○ Change your shampoo every now and then; hair seems to develop a resistance to a shampoo's ingredients after

13

a period of time, sometimes the result of a build-up of styling products. Special shampoos to remove this residue are available.

○ Don't throw away a shampoo that doesn't seem to lather. The amount of lather produced is determined by the active level of detergent used in the shampoo and does not influence its cleansing ability—it is more a cosmetic touch.

RINSE WELL FOR SHINY HAIR

Always rinse your hair thoroughly in clean, warm water to eliminate any remaining shampoo and conditioner. If traces of these are left in the hair they make it look dull and feel sticky, and also leave particles that flake from the scalp like dandruff.

What Affects Your Hair

The physiological well-being of our bodies have direct bearing on the conditioning of our hair. Besides the improper hair-care, there are several other factors that can be detrimental to hair health.

Some of the important factors are mentioned below :

(i) The hair colour and density is greatly determined by hereditary/genes and related causes.

(ii) Reactions of chemicals or drugs you take to cure other ailments.

(iii) Various hormonal changes affecting the body.

(iv) Transmatic experiences and emotional stress. These shall be elaborated when we discuss about hair disorders ahead.

HAIR TYPES AND SCALP CONDITIONS

Normally there are basically three types of hair : oily, dry and normal. In the first type when the oil glands called sebaceous glands in the scalp secrete excess oil, it travels down the hair shaft, causing excessive oiliness on the scalp and hair. The oily

14

hair appears lank, dark and worse. The second type is dry hair. In contrast to the oily hair condition, dry hair is a result of the lack of sebum and oil on the hair causing it to dry out at the cellular level. Flakiness of the scalp and dandruff are a direct result of dryness. The hair books limp, becomes less elastic, growing more and more susceptible to breakage and damage.

The third type is normal hair. It is generally healthy, silky hair without over-dry ends or over-oily roots. It is easiest to cope and care for. But, in any case, this natural gift shouldn't be taken for granted and occasional care must be given to this category as well.

OILY HAIR CARE AND SCALP CONDITIONS

The principle of care for oily hair and scalp condition is no different than taken for oily skin condition.

The whole objective is to remove excess oil and expoliate skin cells which clog up and suffocate the follicles in our scalp. Infection usually erupts in the blocked hair follicles which leads to hair loss and other scalp disorders.

The whole emphasis, hence is laid on cleansing and toning routines. The cleansing routine involves washing and rinsing the hair since the hair has to be washed as frequently as it gets dirty and oily. A natural shampoo on formulation of herbs such as 'Amla' (Emblic Myrobalan) 'Shikakai', Triphala[1] serves the purpose ideally. Remember that an ideal shampoo is always gentle in action, thorough in dissolving the grime and at the same time, not harsh like a detergent shampoo.

As mentioned earlier, massaging hair and scalp is important for the well-being as well as good growth of the hair. For dry hair, scalp massaging with oil is recommended. For oily hair, massage with toning lotion is suitable. A two minutes brushing, stroking and combing routine is sufficient massage exercise for the scalp.

---

1. Three herbal products : Hararh, Baherha, Amla

DESI COSMETIC CARE FOR OILY HAIR

Many people, always ready to spend thousands of rupees on hair-care-might find the home-made solutions quite offensive but the fact can't be denied that the market has till date nothing better to offer-or else Prince Charles wouldn't have been bald in the prime of his youth !

The Recipe

(i) Get some Shikakai powder from the market. Now pound some dried green grams to powder form with fenugreek (Methi) seeds. The proportion should be : 2 : 1 :1 : ½ (Two measures of Shikakai one measure of powdered green grams (flour) and half measure of fenugreek powdered seeds. When required, mix a table spoon of this mixture in the white of an egg and use it as a shampoo. Though it won't lather like a soap or shampoo, it would clean your hair thoroughly.

(ii) Take some 'reetha nuts' (dry soap nuts) and soak them overnight. Mash them in the morning and strain the soapy solutions. Add a teaspoon of Shikakai powder and wash your hair with it.

(iii) A pudina (mint leaves) solution for cleansing your oily hair. This is an infusion recipe. Prepare it and mix it in any shampoo you use. Boil a handful of mint in one- and-half glass of water for 20 minutes. Strain the solution and mix in a 300 ml. bottles of shampoo.

(iv) **Lotion For Toning Your Hair :**
Mix a tablespoon of Malt Vinegar in about 100 gms. of water. Add a pouch of salt in it. Dab two tablespoons of it on your scalp and massage it with your finger tips twice a week. Leave the lotion on for one hour. Rinse with cool water, brush and set your hair.

CARE OF DRY HAIR

Since dry hair tends to be thin and rough, it is more vulnerable to damage and results in split ends.

The whole purpose is to let the hair develop the process of self-lubrication by outside applications. Hence the emphasis on the conditioning aspect of hair-care. Strong cleansing routines and dry touching exercises and massaging of the scalp promote dryness and flakiness of the scalp.

Those with the dry hair should never use strong-action shampoo. Often a generous oil application and massage recommended before washing the hair. Frequent shampooing is also harmful for dry hair. Also, for the moisture-dry hair, a moisturiser application is required.

Two Home-made Recipe of the Shampoo for Dry Hair :

(i) Take a cupful of skimmed milk and beat an egg in it. When the foam becomes consistent, rub it into the scalp have it for 5 minutes. Rinse the hair thoroughly with water. Repeat it twice a weak.

(ii) Mix two tablespoonful of gram flour or one teaspoon of Shikakai in a cupful of coconut milk. Apply this mixture on your scalp and massage your head gently. Rinse it after five minutes. Wash your hair this way at least once a week.

Protein Conditioning Recipe for Dry Hair

A tablespoonful of castor oil should be mixed with one tablespoon of glycerine, a tablespoon of cider vinegar a teaspoon of protein—add to this a tablespoonful mild shampoo (preferably the one recommended for cleansing the infants hair). Apply it on scalp and leave it on for 20 minutes. Rinse with clean water.

A Special Oil for Toning Your Scalp

Take a bottle of good quality castor oil. In case you don't like castor oil, replace it with coconut oil. Add to it a tablespoonful lavender essential oil in it. Heat a little and massage it gently on your scalp at night. Rinse or shampoo it out in the morning. Do so at least thrice a week.

These are all time-tested recipes for toning, cleansing and conditioning of hair.

GENERAL TIPS FOR LOOKING AFTER YOUR HAIR

Conditioner

Conditioners cannot *mend* damaged hair but they can help prevent damage getting worse and protect the hair by leaving a film on the cuticle. They have the effect of flattening the cuticle, which makes light reflect off it so your hair looks wonderfully shiny. Conditioner also works to untangle your hair—especially useful if your hair is over-processed and so tends to be knotty.

○ Use conditioner after every shampoo (on the whole of your head if your hair is dry or just the ends if it is oily)—it shouldn't leave your hair lank unless you do not rinse it properly.

○ Avoid products that claim to shampoo and condition in one because the functions of *washing* and *protecting* are different and cannot really be successfully combined.

○ Apply only a small amount of conditioner as your hair won't absorb any surplus and it will take longer to rinse out.

Drying Without Damage

Let your hair dry naturally as often as possible. With a towel, blot, don't rub the hair. When using a hairdryer point it down the hair shaft to keep the cuticle flat. Do not brush or comb wet hair more than is necessary—it is very vulnerable.

Choosing Combs

When buying a comb, check that it has a smooth join down the centre. Uneven jagged plastic will damage the hair shaft. The best option is a comb that is sawcut in one piece with wide, rounded teeth. Trichologists normally recommend avoiding metal combs which can cause damage.

Care For Long Hair

After washing your hair, don't brush them instantly. Wrap it in a towel and blot out some of the moisture. Rubbing split ends and rubbing very wet hair in its weakened state, pulls out the hair. When your hair is slightly dry, comb it with wide-toothed comb, starting from the ends slowly and working up to the crown. This is the best way to avoid tangles and excessive pulling.

The general problem faced by many is oily scalp, coupled with dry and split ends. In such cases final rinse with diluted hair. Proportion : 1 tablespoon to a mugful of water. This helps restore the acid manth that has just been washed away. Your hair wash should have an application of a good creamy conditioner particularly on the ends.

Those with oily hair must brush repeatedly to keep oil from pooling on the scalp and to carry the oil to hair ends to prevent the problem of end splitting. Split-ends specially in long hair are a result of rough treatment of your hair. Fierced brushing snaps the hair and breaks it off. The use of rubber bands to tie hair together, and bending hair into fish look with metal curlers or rollers can damage your long tresses. Spot baldness in long hair is believed to be a frequent hair problem. Girls with long hair in tight plaits and women who wear a tight chignon are generally the most susceptible victims of this malady. It is always better to keep changing hairstyles to evenly distribute the pulling tension on your hair. Those with long hair who use electric rollers, curbing irons and blow-driers must use the conditioner suiting to them best after shampooing. It helps hair retain the necessary oil and prevent fast drying.

❏

2

Identify The Type of Hair You Have

Although we have thrown in enough hints in the previous chapter to help you identify the type of hair you have, yet more details are thought to be necessary because your hair is your most versatile beauty asset. You can change its style, colour and shape temporarily or permanently which does after your image quite strikingly but what you can't do is change the type of your hair. Since hair-look is quite deceptive and it changes its view as frequently as the season changes, at times people get confused about knowing which type of hair they have. In summers dry and rough look might give you a feeling as if your hair is dry type whereas the fact is that it is due to external conditions. Hence it is extremely important to be aware of your hair types and look after your crowning glory accordingly to keep it in peak condition. The general rule you must remember that beautiful hair is healthy hair, full of bounce and shine.

Recognising your hair type will ensure that you give it the best possible care. There are many factors which will affect your natural hair type and after the needs of your hair. In any case you must fully ensure the type of hair you have or else the foundation will be shaky on which you plan to build your crowning glory.

Although we have mentioned that there are only three types of hair that are generally found, yet since the world going small and marriages between citizens of far different geographical background are becoming common, it is necessary to include more categories. But remember that the remedy suggested or the care hinted for a particular type holds good for that particular type.

DRY AND/OR DAMAGED

The causes of this can be varied :
○ Hereditary.
○ The use of too many harsh chemical treatments, such as bleaching, or incorrect use or over-use of hairdryers or heated rollers.
○ Over-exposure to the sun, sea or chlorinated water.
○ Not using a conditioner.

Hair-Care

○ Shampoo and condition with moisturising products two to three times a week, but if you prefer to wash your hair every day, use a mild shampoo and try a lighter conditioner.
○ Give your hair a deep conditioning treatment once a week.
○ Let your hair dry naturally as often as possible, but if you have to use a hairdryer, set it on a low speed and temperature.
○ Don't use at-home perming or bleaching kits as your hair could become even more damaged—go to a saloon for advice.
○ Wear a bathing cap if you go swimming and a hat, scarf or special hair-protecting product in the sun.
○ Foods high in protein such as fish, poultry and pulses

21

will help combat brittle hair.

○ Massage your scalp gently to improve the circulation and stimulate the sebaceous glands which produce the body's own natural conditioner for hair-sebum.

In case the shampoos and conditioners required for dry hair of your type are not easily available for you, try your desi type-taking the clue from the previous chapter. For example, the shampoo and conditioner suggested earlier could be very effective. You can improvise it a bit, like adding a bit of henna in the solution if you are using the home-made recipe for shampoo or conditioner in summers.

Oily

This can have several causes, including :

○ Heredity.
○ High hormonal activity.
○ Under-or over-washing using harsh products.
○ Brushing too frequently which over-stimulates the sebaceous glands in the scalp.

Hair-Care

○ Use a comb rather than a brush and don't style or touch your hair more than is necessary, to avoid stimulating the sebaceous glands.

○ Use a mild shampoo, washing your hair as often as necessary, and use a conditioner designed for oily hair, but only on the ends.

○ Give your hair a final rinse with a little lemon or vinegar added to the water as this restores the pH balance of your hair.

○ Avoid wearing hats or scarves as they may make the problem worse.

○ Check that your diet is healthy and balanced.

Combination Hair

This combination of greasy scalp with dry ends can be caused by :

○ Chemical treatments such as perming and bleaching.
○ Not having your hair trimmed frequently; approximately every six weeks is usually recommended.

Hair-Care

○ As for oily hair, use a comb in preference to a brush.
○ Shampoo your scalp only; when you rinse out the shampoo it will run down the hair shaft, cleaning it in the process.
○ Try alternating shampoos for dry and greasy hair.
○ Use conditioner only on the ends.

Normal

It is rare to have completely normal hair.

Normal hair is the result of sensible hair-care, regular trims, few, if any, chemical treatments, and a good diet. Oh, and good genes.

Hair-Care

○ Keep to your usual hair-care routine and trims to maintain its good condition.
○ Use conditioner to protect the ends and use an occasional deep-conditioning treatment.
○ Try to avoid damaging your hair with too much chemical processing.

AFRO HAIR

Afro hair has curved follicles, which give it its characteristic springy curl. The hair strands are deceptively thin and are actually fewer in number per square centimetre than other hair types. As a result Afro hair is particularly vulnerable to damage during chemical processes.

Many people with this hair type have their hair straightened, but it is a technically very complicated process and can cause terrible damage to the hair's infrastructure, leading to hair loss unless treated professionally. Do not use at-home straightening kits.

This hair type is invariably dry as its very structure makes it difficult for sebum from the sebaceous glands to travel down the hair shaft.

Hair-Care

○ Massaging a little specially blended hair oil into the hair after shampooing and conditioning helps to alleviate dryness.

○ If you have a mixed hair type, with a greasy scalp and dry ends, avoid using too many oils as they may block the hair follicles. Instead, shampoo minimally and use conditioner only on the ends of your hair, not on the scalp.

○ Braiding looks great on ethnic hair, but you should not keep your hair in this style for long periods, as the constant pulling on the scalp exerts too much pressure on the hair follicles and can lead to hair loss.

Particular Tips

  (i) Don't use detergent shampoos.

 (ii) Regularly massage your scalp.

(iii) First assess whither your scalp and hair are moisture dry or oil-dry.

(iv) Condition your hair as often as you wash it.

 (v) Never comb, brush or massage vigorously if the hair is extremely dry.

Now having conclusively identified your type of hair you have, you read the next chapter which deals with conditioning your hair.

❑

3

How To Condition Your Hair

Not many people realise that our hair is a most hapless victim of pollution that stands over our head especially in the big cities and metropolis like Delhi and Mumbai. As if this is not enough we get dirty and often excessively chlorinated water to wash our hair with. Not only chlorine but other more deadly chemicals may be mixed in that but you feel helpless. And sadly enough that not all. The suffering is worsened by the harsh and strong hair-care with chemical cosmetics, emotional crisis, hormonal problems and adverse weather conditions. All these factors substantially contribute in having our hair split on ends with dryness, limpness, frizziness and its resultant unmanageability to say the least. It is to protect your hair from these hazards to a large extent that a suiting hair conditioner plays its effective role.

Like you have creams and lotion to keep your skin glowing and healthy so you have a hair conditioner for keeping your hair lustrous and shiny. A conditioner can be defined as a beauty preparation that improves texture of the hair and makes them easily manageable. These are generally applied after you have shampooed your hair.

Although many men deem conditioning etc. as exclusively female requirement and they pay scant attention to extending this care to their hair, yet the pressures of modern life have shown how wrong they are. Of course, men pay less attention to their hair since traditionally unkempt hair or baldness has never been considered as bad for them. But now with the advent of various appearance based jobs they have also started realising the importance of proper hair conditioning. It is essential to rejuvenate our hair which is usually robbed of its vitality by the abuse it is exposed to.

You need hair conditioner for two purposes : restoring body and bounce to your limp hair. So there are two kinds of body-building hair conditioners—the ones you rinse out and the ones you leave in. Both work at adding bulk to the hair by leaving some material on the hair shaft which include protein and polymer fibres. The second important reason for going for hair conditioning is its restoring the acid mantle and removing snarls from the hair. There are certain special creamy rinse conditioners that are designed to untangle the snarls in the air. The cream rinse leaves a coat on the hair shaft to help minimise the stress on the hair from brushing, combing, setting and to prevent its breakage and ends getting split. There cream rinses do not add body though they do soften the hair and make it easily manageable.

Often we have our hair damaged due to rough brushing or for other reasons-like sleeping in a wrong posture. Hair conditioning restores the damaged hair into full-bodied hair. The protein in the hair conditioner helps repair the damaged part of the hair.

Sometimes in dry season particularly in winters or in summers when we have to bear direct sun over our heads. The hair conditioners help restore the loss of vital moisture from them due to excessive absorption of heat or getting exposed for long in dry winter.

Of course there are many hair conditioners claiming to make hair bouncy healthy and strong available in the market but first of all their claim is doubtful and secondly they all contain certain chemicals which might temporarily give a shining, healthy look to the hair but in the long run they are found to be damaging. Instead of going for them it is better if you prepare your own hair-conditioners at home. One of them is given below :

26

The material and quantity of it required to prepare your home-made hair conditioner is given below :

Take 1 teaspoonful of each : Castor oil, Amla or Brahmi oil, malt vinegar, glycerine and any mild shampoo. Mix them all to get your desired hair conditioner. While the castor oil would give your hair the body, herbal oil the healthy diet, vinegar works as the catalyst to restore acid mantle, glycerine the much needed moisturising effect and shampoo would play the role of the carrier that takes the other ingredient to their destination. Before washing your hair apply this mixture to the hair gently and leave it for about 20 minutes. Then during both shampoo it out with clear water (lukewarm in winters) to see your hair almost transmogrified in a trice.

Given below the formula of making a hair conditioner for making your hair more shiny and covered with a lustrous sheen. Since this contains onions, may be some of you might not relish the offensive but lingering odour of it but that it is very effective on hair is beyond doubt. Grate few onions and some cabbage together and leave the combination for soaking overnight in a copper vessel. Water should be used as little as possible in fact not more than enough for allowing cabbage and onion pieces to mix well. In the morning add a little of eau-de-cologne to smother the overpowering onion smell. When it smells good, add a few drops of Amla or Brahmi oil. Now apply the mixture and leave it on your scalp for about half an hour. Wash it off with a mild shampoo and feel the superb gloss and shine your looks of hair acquire. Once in a week you can repeat the process to keep your hair healthy and shiny.

Apart from these, other formulae for hair conditioners using henna as the main ingredient have also been in use in the traditional houses which don't succumb to publicity stunt and advertisement tantrums. Two of the most effective old family secrets are being revealed here.

(a) In case your hair is oily, mix 2 tablespoon of yoghurt (or plain curd) and a pinch of sugar to a light paste. Add little water if the paste is thick. Apply it on the hair and leave it on for 20 minutes. Rinse it out with clear water. Shampooing is not recommended. In case you find the smell of yoghurt unbearable, you may use a very mild shampoo to clean your hair.

(b) For dry hair : mix henna in a tablespoon of oil (preferably odourless non-sticky coconut oil) and enough warm milk to make a homogenious paste. Apply and leave it for 20 minutes. Then rinse it out later.

The henna included in it gives hair also a shiny 'tan'. However those who are susceptible to cold should avoid using the yoghurt conditioner in bitter winters. In that time yoghurt may be replaced by malt vinegar.

Apart from these, you can also use a hair conditioner detailed below for only setting your hair. Just take teaspoon of gelatin-easily procurable from the market, in a mug of water. Rinse your hair with it. Dry your hair and set them as you want.

Of course there are many hair-conditioners that are available in the market but see to it which suits you most by trial and error method. In doing so the testing time may be reduced to 5 minutes. Instead of otherwise prescribed 20 minutes. However, our recommendation is that you stick to the home-made ones.

Given below a table to enable you to detect the malady-cause in your hair and treat if immediately.

Malady-Reckoner and the Remedy Table

Hair Condition	Cause	Remedy
Frizzy and uncontrollable	Excessive humidity	Using moisturising cream conditioner.
Limp, flat, brassy	Excessive sweating	Our sweat contains a mild acid which takes out hair's vitality. Add little of coffee powder to your hair conditioner. Rinse and repeat.
Faded, dry	Excessive exposure to sunlight	Wear a hat or use a hair sunscreen.

28

Greenish, brittle	Chlorinated water of the pools you swim in.	Oil massage once a week and soda-water rinse once or twice a week. Always use bathing. Cap while swimming.
Dull, limp, unsettable	Atmospheric pollution	Fight it out with the following solution to rinse your hair with 1 quart water, 2 spoonful rose water, 1 spoon vinegar. Apply rinse out after shampoo twice a month. Keep your hair covered.
Limp and faded	For many reasons especially in hot season.	Use 'Khus-Water' to rinse them after applying your henna based hair conditioner.

❏

$$\boxed{4}$$

Hair Problems

Hair problems appear to multiply with the passage of time. Though it appears so yet it is not the fact. It is only when inadequate treatment gives rise to the other problem with minor variation. We seem to thing as if this is a new problem. Basically there are three major problems that afflict us : dullness, thining and dandruff. These conditions may have several causes and there are a number of different treatments to try.

A. Dull Hair : This could be a temporary as well as a permanent problem. If it is temporary some of the causes you will find in the previous chapter alongwith their possible remedies. In case it appears to be chronic then search its causes among the following reason :

   (a) Stress : Most of the people don't realise that modern life's stresses do play havoc with our hair. Coping with stress automatically restores the shine of the hair. Some of the ideal treatments to deal with this stress problems are : taking yogic exercises, particularly pranayam and medical treatment in consultation with your doctor. He would suggest some exercises and medicine which will clear the stress problem considerably though not fully. In fact, stress can be relieved only by yourself treating you mentally. Of course external distress cannot be eliminated easily but what best you can do is to lessen its impact by altering a bit to your attitude to life. Care for your hair and try to lessen your attitude—you would soon find your hair becoming naturally shining.—

(b) **Not rinsing out Shampoo and Conditioned properly :** This normally happens when you are in hurry to catch your office bus in the morning. In that case it is advisable to devote attention to your hair only in the evening and on Sundays. Always remember to wash your hair clean when you apply shampoo or hair conditioners no matter they be home-made. It is like leaving soap on your body and the skin cracking due to the reaction. If you clean them properly this problem will not trouble your hair.

(c) **A Build-up of the residue of Styling Products :** This is again the cause due to your cleaning or styling up your hair hurriedly. Maybe the product used for styling your hair is not suiting you. Try to see the effect by changing the product or using less of it.

(d) **Sun-Damage :** In a tropical country like India this could be a potential danger for nearly eight to nine months, roughly between March to October. Sometimes during the winters over-exposure to the sun also causes this damage. Which the body might be craving for more heat, the hair has had its fill of heat. Even otherwise when you face the sun keep your head and face always in the shade. It is an old saying in India that always enjoy heat from the fire in the front but from the sun in the back. Moreover, if you have to work in the open for long always use a hat when working under the direct sun. Sometimes the sun rays growing fierce or more deadly by their reaction to the atmospheric pollution may take a heavy tolls of the crown on your head. Be cautious about it, particularly when you don't know what your hair might be receiving with the sun-light following thinning of the Ozone layer. In any case it is always good to keep your head away from the direct sun.

(e) **Heated Drying or Styling Appliances :** The modern age has many electronic gadgets and appliances for doing all sorts of work. Like you have a hair-dryer. In order to dry your hair early without exposing it to the sun we often take resort of the hair dryer and other similar appliances. While occasionally it might be a harmless substitute hair-dryers or various curling appliances regular use take the sheen out of your hair besides weaking them. In fact, this help from modern scientific advancement should be taken sparingly. Avoid styling and drying your hair by any artificial method. Hair-care requires patience and perseverance.

General Treatment for Dull Hair

Rinse with white vinegar after shampooing and before conditioning.

Dry your hair correctly. Read general tips given in the end of the first chapter under the sub-heading 'Drying without damage'. Silicon serums add instant shine. Just apply a few drops to dry hair.

In case your hair appears dull because of residual build-up of the shampoo and hair conditioners, use a mild shampoo like a little of 'beer shampoo' to clean the mess.

Also, avoid chemical treatment until your hair has recovered.

B. Dandruff And Itchy Scalps : Famous western trichologist, Philip Kingsley advises. "Most of us at sometime have a flaky or itchy scalp. The most common cause of itching is dandruff which describes all kinds of scalp flaking. Dandruff is the single most common problem that can occur on everybody. To have a few white-flaked cells is normal for it is simply the sloughing off matured skin cells and waste material through the pores of the scalp. When it becomes excessive it has to be considered as a problem. Well-looked after, clean, healthy hair with the proper acid balance does not have dandruff problem.

As a matter of fact, dandruff is produced when sweat and oil secretions change; the micro-organisms which are controlled by these secretions then multiply, causing the skin on the scalp to be shed faster. Always remember that DANDRUFF IS RARELY THE RESULT OF A DRY SCALP. It is usually oily because the flakes absorb oil. Dandruff and itching can get worse with stress or before menstruation, and can vary with seasons. The foods you eat can also affect the problem. White wine and aspirin may also an itchy scalp. Also, you could be sensitive to your shampoo or conditioner—test this by a process of elimination.

Although anti-dandruff shampoos are quite effective they can often leave the hair too oily, too dry and unmanageable. As an alternative you can ask your chemist to make up a cream containing 1 per cent each of sulphur and salicylic acid. Rub this into your scalp for a few minutes, wash off with your favourite shampoo, then condition. Remember, to keep your hair clean, wash it daily if possible.

In fact, the latest researches prove that there are two forms of dandruff: oily and dry. The dry dandruff appears as loose as white flakes, and the scalp itches. The oily dandruff is sticky and yellow in colour, and the scalp with oily dandruff smells bad. The oily form is found most among adolescents and adults with an excessively oily skin and scalp.

Generally the basic causes of dandruff are faulty diet, emotional tension and stress, hormonal disturbances, infection due to disease, injury to scalp and unwise or excessive use of hair creams lotions etc. Also excessively dry weather may also encourage dandruff.

We might have observed that mostly adolescents have dandruff. It is physiologically a time when they secret an excess of androgen hormones which causes sebum, the skin oil. Hence it is to some extent natural.

The Possible Cures of Dandruff Problem

Besides using special shampoos always remember to keep your hair clean. Wash your hair and scalp frequently—it could be daily or every other day—much depends on how stubborn your dandruff is. In case your hair and scalp are oily, you should use herbal shampoo, since frequent strong shampoo wash can damage your hair.

Apart from other treatments, always remember that massage and daily brushing is extremely helpful in treating dandruff. Both of these hair exercises invigorates the blood circulation to scalp, promote the traffic of oil effusion and dislodge the dead skin cells sticking to the scalp for easy exfoliation. If you have dry dandruff use an oil to massage your scalp especially before washing your hair.

Also, you must devote attention to your diet. Eat less animal fat and more poly-unsaturated vegetable oils. Avoid sweets, chocolates, fried food, shellfish, and excessive intake of iodised salt. Have more of green, leafy vegetables, chicken, fish and its products. You must ensure that your body get an extra dose of vitamins A, E and B complex through your diet. It is better to have your menu-card made for the day and night food.

Some Tried and Tested Formulae for Getting Rid of Dandruff

(i) Shampoo your hair the following way : apply it to the root of the hair by your fingers very softly and massage it gently. Then wash it off with lukewarm water.

(ii) By some 'Triphala' from the market which is easily available there. Mix 1 teaspoon of it in a glass of water and boil. Let it simmer for about three minutes. Cool it strain it and mix with equal quantities of cider vinegar or malt vinegar and massage the lotion in the scalp gently and leave it on. Use the treatment in nights and shampoo next morning. (This treatment is very effective when your dandruff is oily).

(iii) Add to a mugful of water two tablespoons of malt vinegar. After shampoo, rinse the hair with it. Towel-dry your hair. This is an excellent remedy to prevent oily dandruff.

(iv) The following remedy is also very effective on oily dandruff. Soak two spoonful of fenugreek seeds in water overnight. In the morning, make a paste of the seeds and apply on the head. Leave it on for half an hour. Then wash the hair with soapnut (Reetha) or Shikakai and water. You may use a herbal shampoo to wash your hair. Follow this routine at least twice a week.

(v) In case you have dry dandruff, for best results, massage your scalp with one teaspoon of hot castor oil, 1 teaspoon coconut oil and one teaspoon 'til' (sesame) oil. Leave it on for about half-an-hour and then shampoo it out. During winters do so at least twice a week.

(vi) Again, if you have dry dandruff, take about 5 tablespoons of yoghurt (or plain curd) and squeeze half a lime in it. Take two spoonful of green grams and powder them. Mix it in the curd. Apply on scalp and leave it on, for few minutes. Wash your hair with a creamy shampoo suggested earlier. Do so at least twice a week during winters and thrice during summers.

(vii) Take a tablespoon of eau-de-cologne and two aspirins (tablets) crushed into this liquid. Apply it on your hair and wash it off with a creamy shampoo.

(viii) Take a cupful of mild water and squeeze lemon juice into it. Apply on to the roots of your hair and allow it to dry. Do so at least three or four times a week.

(ix) Take a cupful of sour whey (Mattha or lassi) and apply it gently on to the roots of your hair. Then wash it with plain water without using any shampoo. Then rub your hair dry with a soft towel.

(x) Take two spoonful of 'besan' (gram flour without husk). Add a little of plain curd and half a spoonful of lime juice and rub it on your hair roots. Allow it to dry and wash if off with plain water, at least twice a week.

(xi) Never wash your hair with boiling hot water. The extra heat on the scalp encourage dandruff formation.

(xii) Soak overnight Amla and Retha then wash your hair with this water. In winters add a little of hot water to take the chill out of the solution. Wash your hair with this water at least twice a week.

(xiii) Add a little of 'Besan' in a couple of spoonful of vinegar. Then put a few drops of pure honey into it. Quickly apply this paste-like formation on to your hair. Wash it off with a mild shampoo or plain lukewarm water.

(xiv) Rub lukewarm castor oil on to your hair. Then soak a soft towel in hot water and squeeze the water out of it. Cover your head with this towel and keep your head covered this way for about 10 to 15 minutes. Then remove the towel and wash your head with lukewarm (or cold) water. This indirect fomentation will immediately help hair gain strength and fight against the itchy flakes.

(xv) Take a little of Besan and make the solution by adding to the sour whey. Rub this lotion gently in your scalp and covering your head with a towel stay as you are. Then wash your hair with cold or lukewarm water depending upon the season.

(xvi) Take the leaves of Mehndi (henna) and boil them with Amla, Shikakai and Baherha (of fruit of the tree Belleric myrobalan) and a little of water for about 10 minutes. Then cool the solution, mesh the fruity ingredients and strain. Apply this water on to the root of your hair then let it soak for half an hour. Wash it off with cold water in summers and with lukewarm water in winters. This is a very effective treatment to get rid of all kinds of dandruff problem.

(xvii) Normally if you rinse your hair with a little of vinegar (diluted with water) solution every time you clean your hair, you might never face this dandruff problem.

In case the dandruff does not clear up in time you should take medical advice. At times persistent dandruff problem could be the consequence of a fungal infection.

C. Falling Hair or Thinning Hair : Thinning hair and hairloss can be caused by following reasons :

Stress, Hormonal Changes, Poor diet.

Pulling the hair while brushing or scrapping it back too often into light pony tails. Most of these reasons have been elaborated on in the earlier pages. Even the dietary part has been discussed while diciphering the reasons behind excessive formation of dandruff. But apart from these factors it must also be made clear-that hair, like human beings, has a life style. Every hair that grows must fall out one day. New hair will grow at the place after sometime.

A natural query is as to why this natural phenomenon be reckoned as a problem. Indeed, why ? Is it not akin to the population control problem. When all those who are born must die, why must the population increase ? In fact, all these queries have one single answer : they are counted in the particular period of time. We are not dealing with the problem of eternal nature. It is confined to a span of 70 or 60 or a maximum hundred years. Hence what is true with the number of people in a country in a given span of time, so is also true for hair on a particular head !

But we must appreciate that there is a natural balance between the rate at which hair falls and the rate at which new hair grows. Any disturbance in this balance can result in an excessive fall of hair or hair all over the body.

Now a days this problem of hair-loss seems to be getting magnified, ironically, despite many cures being suggested helped, aided and abetted by modern gadgetry. The problem of hair-loss happens for various reasons such as emotional and physical stress of modern life, local scalp infection, adverse drug reaction, hormonal imbalances during teenage, pregnancy etc. apart from some special reasons like hereditary factor also.

37

Main Culprits

The dermatologists, over past few decades have made some interesting findings that, to a greater degree of cogent reasoning, explain the pattern of hair loss. It has been found to be provenly related to the rate of hair growth, length of the hair, age and even the pigment that imparts particular colour to hair. It has been, therefore, estimated that it is normal to shed 70 to 8 hair a day and it is normal for each of those hair to be replaced by the hard working follicles. It has also been calculated that on any given day about 80 to 90 per cent hair are in the growing stage. This period roughly lasts about 1000 days and 10 per cent hair are in the resting stage which continues for about 100 days before the eventual growing out of the follicles. It has also been noticed that a male showing his facial hair growth every morning so the head hair fall-out occurs monthly. Although why hair die out in the morning is not yet scientifically explained yet the most plausible explanation is that hair being a biological product completes its cycle-or its 'check-out' time is also morning. Curiously enough, it has been estimated that longer the hair the lesser is the fall-out. The studies revealed that on an average the four in long hair lose as many as 70 to 80 strands a day while 12-inch long hair-20 to 30 strands and 20-inch long as little as 10 to 16 hair a day. Hence the conclusion is shorter the hair-the greater is the hair loss.

The normal growth-rate of hair is estimated to be about 5 to 6 inches a year and shortfall in the normal hair growth is accompanied with a hair loss also. Besides, there are distinct stages when the hair loss is believed to be more than usual. These are : birth to three years, at three and 10 years, at 10 and 25 years, at 30 and 55. It is believed that the hormonal changes in the body has a direct bearing on the hair loss. In case of women the maximum hair growth occurs between 15 to 30 again on account of hormonal changes since growth of estrogen is believed to promote hair growth. Perhaps this hormone's presence in the body accounts for the reason as to why there are hardly bald women. Another reason could be that since women keep longer hair on an average than men in the latter case the hair-loss is significantly less. Perhaps due to the principle mentioned earlier that the longer the hair the lesser the hair-loss. Still when man keeps long hair they do become bald. In fact, the mysteries of hair have not yet been finally exploded. Hopefully with the future research work would unveil this mystery as also find the means to prevent hair-loss. At present, suffice it to say that if you keep your scalp clear, hair long and free of dandruff you have every chance of keeping your pats fully covered with lustrous and bush hair growth.

What Causes the Excessive Hair-loss or Baldness

Of course we shall be discussing baldness later on but here we are elaborating on the intermediatory stage.

In medical terminology, temporary or permanent hair loss to an excessive degree is defined by the disorder called ALOPECIA. The cause of baldness or hair-loss is due to many factors line

(i) **Hereditary :** It is the genes we inherit that generally determine the kind of hair we have : curly, straight, thin, thick, fine, sparse, dark brown, black or blonde. This hereditary factor is greatly responsible for your hair-growth as well although your especial care can always prolong the life of your hair. Generally the problems of concerning hair-loss are also passed on from the parents to the offspring. It has been found that disorders related with thyroid deficiency and diabetes also adversely affect the life of hair. Of course there are other diseases as well like typhoid which cause much hair-loss but that is only a temporary phase. The major threat to healthy hair comes from diabetes and thyroid disorders. However, the basic genetic cause of the hair-loss is hereditary. But there is no doubt that with assiduous care of hair you can easily prolong the life span of the hair.

(ii) **Stress Factor and Trauma :** Medically 'Traction

Alopecia' is the term employed to describe the effect on the hair due to stress or trauma. In ladies case this can be caused by tying up the hair in too tight 'Chignon Style', ponytails and pigtails. If the hair are kept stretched for a prolonged duration, the constant pull-like pressure on the hair can result in spot baldness. Also a sudden shock experienced due to some traumatic or highly disturbing news can also lead to spot baldness. It is believed that Shahjehan, the famous Mughal Emperor, lost his hair when his beloved Mumtaj Mahal expired suddenly. Also a severe blow to head may lead to spot baldness where the blow is received. Generally a severe blow on the head makes the portion of the head-at least Cranium—much with follicles rendered inactive. In that case the baldness is unavoidable because how the hair will grow over dead cells ?

Head Infection : There are many bacterial, viral or fungal infections that can cause hair-loss, though it is a temporary effect and with the cure of infection hair can regrow at that spot.

Hair-Loss Due to High Fever Inducing Disease : Increase in body temperature consistently for a long period adversely affects the hair. Some internal disorders and infections which cause high fever such as flu, pneumonia and typhoid are often accompanied by excessive hair-loss but what is a redeeming feature is that this loss is temporary in most of the cases. Soon after recovery, as the body regains its normal health the hair reappears unless other factors also join—like any of the factors mentioned above.

In Reaction to Certain Drugs and Chemicals

Most of the antibiotics cast an adverse effect on the hair. It is because the theory of antibiotic treatment stands on the premises that the best way to fight against any infection is to resist the body growth. Hence the name 'anti-biotics'. 'Bio'–we all know-means life and anti means against. So the very name suggests it to be against life-growth. The idea is that since infection also grows in the body by drawing strength from the body, if body's growth is temporarily checked, owing to not getting any diet the infection would automatically die down. The point here is not whether this system of treatment is good or not but does this theory adversely affect hair too ? The answer is very much yes. Obviously when the body growth is resisted the hair will also be deprived of their stable diet. There are also some drugs besides anti-biotic medicines like cortizone which are administered sometimes in treating acne and scars also lead to hair-loss. Chemical therapies given in serious diseases such as cancer also cause excessive hair-loss and, at times, even total baldness.

Environmental Stress : Some people are unable to cope with pressures of life. They keep on worrying since they find their problems not heading towards solution. This sets in a sort of permanent stress in their minds, making it 'addicted' to worrying and at times, even 'inventing' worries. With the tension in their minds, the muscles of the scalp always remain constrict, so of the neck, impeding the blood circulation in the process. When blood doesn't reach properly to the root of the hair, the hair weaken consequently. Thus those who believe in remaining serious and sombre with the 'stiff upper lip' should always remember that this they do at the cost of their hair. No wonder the strong protagonist of this demeanour, the Englishmen suffer maximum hair-loss.

This explanation also explains inadvertently the reason as to why ladies have comparatively much less hair-loss than gentlemen. Because not that they have much less, even otherwise to obstruct the flow of blood :

(i) their tension bearing capacity is much less than their husbands. Whenever tension accumulates in large measure their saturation point is reached which sets in other process—triggering the tear-cells to wash off their tension with the stream of tears. All this boils down to the basic truth: keep smiling and tension-free if you want to keep your hair lustrous and shining.

41

Hair-loss Due to Hormonal Imbalance

It is almost the primary cause (only probably second to the hereditary factor) is hormonal imbalance. Pregnancy, contraception with birth control pills and menopause are the common conditions that induce hormonal changes which have been elaborated on below.

(a) **Pregnancy :** This is an inescapable ordeal through which every aspiring mother has to pass. Since motherhood is believed to be the acne of womanhood only the most unfortunate ones are deprived of this privilege. Initially the onset of pregnancy improves the hair condition tremendously as the endocrinal glands functions peaks during this process only. The hair-loss starts only after the birth of the baby due to general enervation of the system and also due to irregularity in the function of the thyroid glands. The normal hair loss after delivery happens four months after the birth and continues for about two months. During this period the lady must take extreme care of her hair and if the hair loss is more then the doctor or trichologist should be consulted. In normal case the precautions as suggested earlier for hair-care should be taken.

(b) **Birth Control Pills :** These pills also cause hormonal imbalance in the body. However, ironically, if a woman in perfect health with normal weight having regular periods, eating normally and physically active, takes the pill for contraceptive reason, this problem of hair-loss does surface, whereas a woman who is already suffering from hormonal imbalance takes the pill, she will find her hair growing more thick since the hormonal imbalance is checked. Hence you would have to find which category you are in.

(c) **Menopause :** As we all know at this stage the female hormone estrogen's production is considerably slowed down, resulting in weak, dry hair and excessive fall out in fifty per cent cases. In case you find your hair-loss quite alarming, consulting the trichologist is a must.

Since these are almost inevitable stages for women, every woman has to cope with them with due care and attention to her hair. Although hair-loss does increase at these stages, there have been instances when growth of hair gets a shot with the menopause. It happens in generally those women case who have not conceived.

How to Cope with These Inevitable Conditions

The normally healthy hair also falls but since they are quickly replenished by the fresh hair growth, the loss does not appear alarming. Generally the hair loss is more in rainy season when the conditions are wet and we know a wet hair becomes weak. In the period following the season of rains almost immediately after it—they become again strong. The growth of hair is best during December to April. The excess fall-out of hair occurs mostly in extreme conditions. A general percentage for all persons is to never comb your hair when they are wet or too dry.

It is by taking especial care through conditioning and nourishing the hair that the hair-loss can be prevented. Cream rinses help the dry and rough hair to regain its flexibility. Generous application of moisturisers and oil preparations replenish the moisture and oil in the dry hair. In this context remember that you should never use other's comb or brush to set your hair.

To control excess fall-out of hair a very important element is massage. Massaging invigorates the blood circulation, giving hair an increased supply of nutrition and oxygen for healthy growth. Massage also stimulates the dormant hair follicles to grow fresh hair. Those with oily skin should avoid using thick oil for the massage. It is better to use light and non-sticky oil which is now easily available in the market. Apart from general massage try the following home-made lotions and cream to prevent the hair-loss. These age-old recipes have withstood the test of time.

(a) **Seeds' Paste :** Take about four to five grams of black-pepper and equal amount of lime seeds. Take about a spoonful of freshly extracted ginger juice and grind the seeds of lemon and black-pepper in this fluid. In case ginger juice is not available you can substitute the same with plain cold water. It is better to dry grind the seeds and then add the ginger juice or water to that powder to make a smooth paste. Apply this paste every night on your head. Leave it for about a couple of hours if you can't bear the paste whole night on your head. This should be applied with the finger tips gently on root of the hair. You may wash it that very night or early in the morning. Try to massage your scalp with soft hands while applying the paste. Wash it off with lukewarm water. This paste would rejuvenate your hair. What is odd is the tingling sensation you feel after applying the paste which many find unbearable. In that case, it is better to apply this paste early in the morning as you get up, leave it on while finishing your morning chores. Make more that the paste remains at least two hours on your head before you wash it.

(b) **Paste for Spot Baldness :** This is also a very efficacious paste to cure spot-baldness. This spot-baldness could result owing to many reasons : the beginning of the effect of infection, accidental pulling of the hair of particular region and like. To make this paste take a few small sticks of Mulathi (liquorice) in milk cream. Add a little of saffron (Kesar) and apply the combination on the bald patch at night. The minimum time it should remain on your scalp is at least three hours. You can apply in the night or early in the morning. Wash it off with clear water in the morning. Some people add Dhatura (seeds) or the fruits of 'Datura alba' which is a powerful narcotic to increase the potency of the remedy. Massage your bald scalp generously with finger tips for five minutes while applying the ointment. This is almost a magic treatment to cure spot baldness.

Even total baldness can be controlled by this treatment, although to some this might create an allergic effect. So before going in for it, it is better to test it before hand like you test the hair-dyes-apply a little on the back of the ear and see its effect in twenty four hours. If you find any adverse effect, remove some of the allergy-causing ingredients like Dhatura.

(c) Take a handful of black-tipped green chillies. These chillies are very pungent and generally grown in the hilly regions. Grind them to a paste form and apply the same on your bald patch a little. This may cause a very unpleasant burning sensation. Wash it with cold water after 15 minutes. While washing it make sure that the paste doesn't enter your eyes for this might cause even blindness. It is advisable to rub a little of coconut oil once you have washed the spot.

(d) **An Efficacious Oil Massage :** The ingredient containing white iodine is believed to be very effective to restore lost hair. Castor oil is a rich source of that. Make sure that you get only pure form of castor oil without containing any adulteration. Most of the castor oil available contain perfumes. These perfumes often lessen the potency of white iodine. Hence massage your hair always with pure castor oil if you want to control your hair-loss. This oil is to be applied with pieces of cotton. Part your hair in small sections and apply the oil with the help of cotton piece at the hair roots or at the bald-patch. Massage it with your tips. If you are able to get white iodine solution, apply it the some way on alternate dry.

Another good massage lotion is prepared the following way. Squeeze the milk out of half a coconut shell. Mix it with the juice of half a lime and massage the solution in your scalp with finger tips but with a vigorous stroke. Make sure that your vigorous massage doesn't uproot the strands. The ideal way is to apply the solution on your finger tips and rub it in your scalp. Leave it for 6 to 8 hours and wash it off with a mild shampoo.

A solution of ground fenugreek seeds, the crushed hibiscus leaves and a spoonful of mild shampoo should be mixed together to form a thick paste. Apply this paste on your scalp and leave it for 4 to 6 hours. Then wash it off with clear water. Instead of shampoo you can also use 'Reetha' solution since shampoo or the Reetha solution performs the duty of a carrier. It makes the Hibiscus leaves and fenugreek seeds essence to the hair root. Wash it off with water. Then you need not use any shampoo since the shampoo or Reetha solution already mixed in the lotion would automatically ease your washing operations. The following precautions you must take if you want to ensure no hair-loss or the onset of baldness.

(i) First check which is the primary cause of your thinning hair or baldness. If it is due to fungal, viral or bacterial infections always consult a registered dermatologist instead of rushing in for instant cures. Otherwise your impatience might aggravate the problem. If the cause is not any infection, you can start the home-made lotions' application as suggested on the previous pages.

(ii) As hinted earlier, make sure that you are not using other's combs or brushes or not allowing them to use your own. People don't realise that most of these infections are contagious. Sanitize your implements i.e., brushes, combs or twirling apparatus etc. at least once a week.

(iii) In case you are affected with spondylitis, it might also cause hair loss since the blood circulation gets affected. In that case never use high pillow.

(iv) Always use a soft brush with well-spaced bristles. In case you use the comb, the ideal one is made of ivory. Its bristles should be sharp enough to cause a mildly incisive sensation on your scalp but not hard enough to wound your scalp which you are combing.

(v) Regular intake of carrot juice (a cupful) to which half a lemon's juice has been added is a very good oral tonic for the hair. This is also called Brewer's Yeast.

(vi) Sometimes lack of iron in the blood or low haemoglobin

count also cause hair-loss. Have your blood tested. If you find it less than 10% it means that your blood needs external supply of iron to make good the deficiency. Consult your doctor and start taking iron tablets.

(vii) Reduce carbohydrate intake (like potatoes, rice etc.) and add more protein to your diet. Remember that obesity and bush hair are generally not compatible. Very rarely you would come across-at least in India- a fat and flabby person who is not bald. The reverse is also true. Extra intake of carbohydrates not only enhances your growth, it also disturbs the good hair growth. Of course a discussion with your dietician might come healthy but if you don't have a week system enhance the protein content of your diet.

(viii) If you are pregnant, approaching your menopause or regularly taking the pills for contraceptive reasons and you find your hair-loss increasing, consult your physician first.

In any cause, like in any other case, if you have hit upon the correct diagnosis you might also get the right cure of your malady for, unless it is well determined by observing the physical characteristics and studying the other causes for hair-loss, the treatment given in previous pages might not prove effective. On the contrary, it might aggravate the situation. Hence seeking the professional help is always better.

Hair represents—like nails—the continuity of life in death. The fallen hair is dead; the cut nail is also dead: though in itself both might represent the symptom of life, they are essentially dead objects. Unlike skin, in itself they might not react, but till they are on your body they need full care.

❑

5

Some More Solutions to The Hair Problems

Although for typical hair problems we have already given the solutions. The following solutions are good for all types of hair whether on a male or a female head.

(i) For dry and dandruff hair the standard treatment is : massage your hair with the lotion made from lukewarm water, coconut and castor oil, mixed in even quantity. After the massage keep your hair covered with a towel soaked in hot water so that the steam fomentation be possible. Then apply half a spoonful of fresh lime juice at the root of the hair. Then after half an hour shampoo your hair and rinse it out with clear water. A fortnight of this treatment would clear out dandruff and make your hair lustrous and soft.

(ii) To prevent the hair-loss (particularly males) should try the following treatments.

Steam your hair at least twice a week. The proper way of steaming them is to cover your head with a hot towel or expose your head to steam rising from the boiled water.

After your bath, add 4 spoonful of vinegar in the water and rinse your hair with it. When your hair has dried rub vinegar again on your scalp, precisely at hair-roots. This precaution checks hair-loss considerably.

An age-old remedy is using til-seeds (sesame and its products) at least during winters. This treatment makes your hair silky, dense, soft and long.

(iii) A pregnant woman must consume at least one piece of Murabba of Amla every day to check hair-loss due to hormonal changes.

(iv) Boil a good quantity of Neem and Ber (a kind of berry fruit available in winters) leaves in a jugful of water. Wash your hair with this concoction after straining and cooling it. This is also a very effective remedy.

(v) Take the leaves of Basil (Tulsi), soak them overnight in water and then grind the soaked leaves and dried and crushed Amla fruit. Now add their concoction in a bucketful of water and wash your hair with this water. This also helps in effectively checking the hair loss. But you must ensure that this water does not enter your eyes as it would cause irritation and might also damage your eye-sight.

(vi) Take a handful of green Amla fruits, grind their pulp to a paste form and apply this pulp to the root of your hair. This remedy not only checks the hair-loss but also strengthens the root of hair. Wash the paste off with a mild shampoo only when it has dried.

(vii) Take about five or six Nimbolis (the yellow fruit of the Neem trees). Grind their pulp and apply the same to the root of your hair to provide them strength.

Henna : An Effective Hair conditioner and Tonic

For centuries together Henna or Mehndi has been used as an effective hair conditioner for strengthening your hair. Since it leaves a cold-effect on the head only during extreme winters its use should be avoided. Otherwise with every hair remedy if you want you can add a little of henna for still better effect. During the summers a paste of henna leaves kept on the head, not only fortifies hair but also cures the boils and blisters developing on the scalp. It is also an ideal remedy to cure headache due to extreme heat.

(i) If you have your hair dry with split ends, and unhealthy looking, prepare the solution in the following way.

Take about 10 gms. henna powder, half a cup castor oil and two big spoonfuls of lime juice and put them in a big jar to let them marinate for about couple of days. Then take out this solution and apply them on the scalp, hair roots and at full length of hair. Then massage your hair vigorously. After the massage wear a plastic cap on your head and cover the cap also with a hot napkin. Allowing this kind of indirect fomentation for about half an hour, wash the lotion off with some mild shampoo. Although this might appear a very cumbersome remedy it has been found to be very effective. Do so twice or thrice a month to have your hair lustrous, soft and silky.

(ii) To check hair-loss, mix a little juice of Kateri (a herb) with henna powder and honey and apply the lotion on the spot baldness at least twice a week. You will soon find the new hair sprouting.

GENERAL GUIDELINES ABOUT HAIR-CARE

Never change your shampoo brand. Once you have seen that a particular brand of shampoo is taking adequate care of your hair, stick to it. Also don't get confused if you find your shampoo is not generating enough lather. Lather is generated by the effect of chemicals with water and it has not much role to play in cleaning your hair. Always untangle your hair with the help of a brush or comb before shampooing them. This way your hair won't be uprooted in large numbers. Shampoo your hair gradually in the same way as you massage your head. Take a little-preferably diluted solution-of shampoo and apply at the hair roots with the tip of your hands. First apply on the scalp and then on the strand of the hair. Never vigorously rub it on the hair. Before shampooing wetten your hair a bit since it helps in the proper application of the shampoo on your scalp.

Use the conditioner always after shampooing your hair. The following home-made conditioner is very effective. Take yellow part of two eggs and beat it thoroughly with warm water. Now rub it gently on your scalp. Wear a cap and let it remain for 10 minutes. Then wash it off with warm water. You will find your hair lustrous and untangled by this kind of post-shampoo operation.

For oily hair always apply a little of lime juice as a hair conditioner and then wash it off with cold water. In case you have oily hair remove fried, roasted items from your menu and supplant them by more of egg, meat, fish, paneer, salad, fruits and green and leafy vegetables.

In case you are too hury to use hair conditioners available in the market or produced at home, the best way you can get rid of the extra oil from your hair by adding just a spoonful of boric powder in a bucket and rinse your hair finally with that water. To treat your extra dry-hair occasionally putting olive oil on to your scalp and massaging it gently with your finger tops might help. Then wash it off with a mild shampoo.

Never use strong hair spray since it puts extra dryness into your hair due to the effect of the chemical inside it.

Nowadays in a big city like Delhi, the non-availability of sweet water tends to make your hair extra dry. Occasional massage with non-sticky and unperfumed coconut oil might prove handy to keep your hair free of the extra-dryness. After you have massaged the coconut oil on your scalp wait for two hours and wash it off with the following lotion made from Shikakai. Boil Shikakai and water 1 : 6 ratio. When the beans of Shikakai are fully melted in the heat allow them to cool. Then mesh the beans with your hands and strain the concoction. Wash your hair with this solution instead of using any shampoo or soap. This would surely reduce the dryness in the hair.

51

For dry hair try another simple recipe : Take a big piece of Multani Mitti (a kind of soft clay, easily available in the market) and soak it in a cupful of water. When it is fully dissolved add a little of coconut oil to prepare a soft dough of the two. Rub it gently in your scalp, allow it to dry and wash it off with clear water. Multani Mitti is also very effective in cooling your head even otherwise. In fact it is a standard prescription in naturopathic treatment to eliminate heat in the head due to environmental heat. This is very good for hair as well. Yet another simple remedy to treat your dry hair is : beat a fresh egg with a spoonful of fresh lime juice and equal quantity of coconut oil. Rub this solution for half an hour on your scalp. Then rub the Shikakai solution suggested earlier and wash it off with an extremely diluted vinegar plus lime juice solution. Such persons must take care to protect their hair from direct sun-rays.

The problem that often disturbs those with mixed type of hair-like dry at the bottom but oily at the top which appear very lustrous after shampooing. Any treatment of one type of hair damages the other type. In this case wash your hair quickly with Shikakai or shampoo as soon as you feel itching sensation. Let shampoo be rubbed only at the top of the strands and not at their bottom level. Persons with such type must always keep their hair clean.

Special Care For Curly Hair

Curly hair is always difficult to mould in the desired shape. If you have curly hair, make sure that you brush them several times a day. Massage lukewarm coconut oil into the roots of the hair from bottom to top. This will help your hair to straighten them out. Develop a habit of combing or brushing your hair after you have wettened the comb or the brush. Tie your curly hair always tightly. This is a long-drawn process to straighten your curly hair or reduce its curl to a great extent permanently.

Every week 'press' your hair with the electric press. Ask your friend or close relation to move lightly hot iron press on your hair. For this you will have to low yourself so that your hair is evenly spread on the press-table. Using big rollers the reverse way is also effective. But use the rollers very sparingly as their regular use weaken hair.

Make sure that you don't rub your hair roots vigorously while washing it.

Greying of Hair and Lice Problem

Untimely greying of hair is a problem that has, become rampant. Now even young lads of 17-18 face this problem which used to afflict only at the middle age. Greying of hair, in fact, takes away the entire charm of a person in old age.

There are many reasons for this problem. Hereditary factor, sudden trauma and the lack of Vitamin 'A' and 'D' are some of the major factors that give rise to this problem. Of course you have numerous dyes now available in the market but that is, in fact, no solution to the problem. It is like finding an escapist's cover to the problem.

Given below is an effective cure for this hair problem. Take a 100 gm of castor oil, 1 ounce sandal powder and even amount of coffee seeds' powder. Heat all the three for about 20 minutes. When it is cold, strain and fill it up in a clean bottle. Massage this hair every night on your scalp and wash your hair early in the morning. This would not only turn your grey hair into black but also prevent the greying of hair.

Another hair lotion to keep your hair black is the following : Take a spoonful of henna powder and equal amount of dry Amla and tea leaves. Put these ingredients into a cupful of hot water. Now add 1/4 spoonful of salt and 1/2 spoonful of rosewater. On the top of it mix two spoonful of fresh lime juice. Let this solution lie as it is for about 5 hours, then start applying in the root of the hair. Leave the solution for about two hours. Just use this twice a week to keep your hair dark and lustrous.

Lice Problem : Lice and tiny lice (called 'Leekhen') in common parlance, problem is hardly paid any attention in these kind of books. Nevertheless it is a bitter problem particularly with the long hair. Hence its victims are generally the girls. But gradually these problems have also started troubling the male folks.

About lice one thing is very clear. Their breeding ground is always the filth that gets accumulated if the hair are not combed frequently. You must remember that combing or brushing of the hair is not wanted only for setting your hair right but also for giving your hair a much-needed massage and brushing out the filth gathering on them. Hence the first and foremost step of getting rid of these lice is to comb your hair frequently and before you retire for the day, vigorously.

Some other tried and tested remedies to get over this problem are given below :

  (i)   Add a bit of camphor to your coconut hair and massage your hair frequently with this solution. Every time you do so you should add a fresh piece of camphor to your coconut oil. Keeping camphor mixed coconut oil for long duration would nullify the camphorial effect. Also, make sure that the coconut oil you choose is odourless and non-sticky one. Sticky one will attract more dirt from the atmosphere which odour will tend to nullify the effect of camphor. After massaging your hair with camphor-mixed coconut oil, wash them with Retha or Retha based shampoo. In the final rinse add a spoonful of dettol or savlon in a mugful of clear water and give a final wash to your hair with this solution. This will also take care of the boils etc. growing on the hair in dry cold and hot summer months.

 (ii)   Add a little oil with black pepper powder and massage this on your scalp. Then after 10 to 15 minutes comb your hair vigorously with a metal comb—iron combs for this purpose are ideal which are easily available in the market. The teeth of this iron comb should be very closely placed.

(iii)   There are now a variety of anti-lice lotions and creams that are now available in the market. Apply a little of them on your hair then cover your hair with a light cloth and retire. In the morning remove the cloth and wash your hair with a mild shampoo. You would find them washed away after your bath. But don't get complacent on our cleaning; repeat the medicine after a week or ten days. It is only when you find your scalp free of lice that you should stop the treatment. Even then occasional medicinal wash at least in rainy season and cold winters would be necessary to finally liberate yourself from the menace of lice.

Problems of Boils and Split-End Hair

Generally during winters owing to extreme dryness of the atmosphere you develop boils. Sometimes they also develop when you are exposed to direct heat of the sun. In either case the best remedy—already explained in the previous pages—rinse your hair finally with a weak antiseptic solution. Any antiseptic solution like dettol or savlon will do. If you have plenty of Neem trees around your house, pluck a few soft leaves of Neem, boil them in a mugful of water, cool, strain and finally rinse your hair with this solution.

Normally people with high blood sugar level get troubled by boils and blisters. In case you find this problem recurring have your blood sugar also checked. In case you find it more than the optimum level, consult your doctor. Once the sugar problem is controlled boils problem will automatically be taken care of. In any case, keep your hair clean and free of lice and filth. An occasional massage with olive oil and coconut oil mixed solution would also control this problem. Remember that boils normally occur when your scalp is not getting clean air—perhaps due to the obstructions caused by the accumulated filth.

Split-end Hair Problem : In case you have more such hair it is better to cut them from the point the strands get split up. In fact, it is better if they are lacked off half an inch before they split. This would prevent the strands getting divided into two parts. Otherwise if you leave the problem as it is you might find the strands getting divided up to their very roots. This precaution will also help you check the hair-loss since when the hair is split up into two strands it weakens the strength of the hair.

In order to get permanent cure of this problem in winters

55

a massage with pure Almond oil and in summers with pure and non-sticky type coconut oil is essential following the massage-at least for 10 minutes. You must comb your hair blunt-edged. Incisive teeth of the comb normally give rise to the problem of hair with split-ends. In case you prefer to comb your hair with brush make sure its bristles are not sharp-edged. Also never comb your hair with a brush having synthetic bristles.

Hair Problems and Acupressure Treatment

The belief of the acupressure therapy rests on the conviction that there are certain points on your body which if pressurised in a special way cure many problems afflicting you. Since the origin of this therapy, China gives great significance to human hair, no wonder this therapy has some vital guidelines to keep your hair shining and lustrous. It believes that the hair is not a dead object and its health and glow is reflective of your overall good health.

Acupressure believes that our nails and hair have a deep relationship. Hence it suggests that you must rub your hand nails with each other twice or thrice in a day with each rubbing lasting for five to six minutes which will not only prevent the hair-loss, untimely greying of hair, dandruff and other conditions but will also keep your hair healthy and shining naturally. In Buffer-Hand Reflexology, an authority on Acupressure, Dr. (Mrs.) Mildred Carter advises : "rub the finger nails of one hand directly across the finger nails of the other hand with a quick, rapid motion as though you were buffing them with a buffer and only you are using the finger nails of the opposite hand as the buffer."

Apart from it if you want to ensure good hair put occasional pressure upon your thumb and big toes from your other hand's index and thumb. The pressure must be applied all around the thumb with one hand. Then repeat the process with other hand. Since the thumb is supposed to control the head region of your body by acupressure theories, pressure on it—twice or thrice a week-would keep your hair healthy and lustrous.

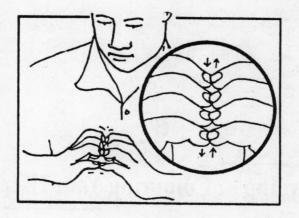

Acupressure also suggests mild winter sun: fomentation on your hair as necessary to prevent the hair loss.

❑

6

Dyeing or Colouring Your Hair

Looking old when you are young is what no sane man or woman would like. But when the indication from your top starts bearing such unpleasant signals it is time you should care about it. It is because grey hair on one's head does not necessarily mean advancing age since white or grey hair now can show their presence even in the teens or twenties. Of course depending upon their gene formation there might still be some people having their hair as black as root even in the eighties. Greying hair just means that the body has stopped making colour pigment. But it is a slow process since no body can grow overnight. Even-though shock or illness may affect production of pigment it is not until the new hair has grown that you see it as white. Hence a piece of advice for those of you who do not colour their hair. They should choose softer colours in cloth and make up, since the skin colouring is also toned down by the same natural ageing process. There is a theory that claims that hair-colouring also gives a pick to your scalp-skin cells which sends a sympathetic wave all over the body to improve your skin texture. Though it appears rather far fetched yet the fact is that dyeing your hair does give it a new pick of buoyancy and body provided you have used the right kind of dye.

HOW TO GO ABOUT IT

Colouring is one of the quickest warp to change your image. Check out all the options to find the best method for your skin. Before you make any changes to the colour of your hair, think about your colouring, features, age and even your occupation. Remember too, that what looks great on someone else may not suit you.

It's a good idea to try on a few wigs in colours and styles that you are thinking of—particularly if you are contemplating a dramatic change. Alternatively, some salons have a specialized computer that can show you images of yourself with different tones in your hair.

If you want a more permanent colour change, rather than just a rinse, go to a salon. An expert colourist will examine your hair and make *realistic* suggestions, taking your hair's health, porosity and natural colour into consideration, as hair colours react differently on various types and conditions of hair.

There are several different colouring techniques. Listed below are the most commonly used, what they do and how long they last. However colouring technology is advancing so much year by year, it's worth asking your local salon what they have to offer.

Colourways

For the most natural-looking effects, just choose a shade or two lighter or darker than your natural hair colour.

Temporary Colour rinses

The hair shaft is coated with colour to darken or highlight it in this treatment. These colour the hair by coating the cuticle and wash out quickly. They normally shampoo-in, but you can buy them in the form of setting lotions. In case you are not going to fight the white, the temporary rinse will keep it looking bright. It is really temporary rinse, coating each hair only until the next shampoo. Colours come in coloured conditioning setting lotions which will enhance white hair with silver pearl or three colours.

59

Although rinse can be used on all non-processed hair, they work best on fair hair. A rinse can also add brownish gold or copper highlights to light or medium-coloured hair. It can bring out the red in the hair and brighten your dark hair with shine. They are cheap, quick and easy to use at home.

Semi-Permanent Colour : They, logically, are not as permanent as a tint, but more lasting than a rinse, penetrating the cuticle only.

Like rinses, semi-permanent colours don't produce a dramatic change unless you choose a dark shade. They penetrate the hair slightly and don't require the aid of a peroxide developer. The hair colour produced by such products fades gradually and naturally, lasting through four to six shampoos. As the colour fades there is no root retouching to do. But most semi-permanent colouring will only hide up to 25 percent grey. They blend white hairs into your normal shade, but usually don't cover them completely. The secret of success is to choose a colour as near as your own as possible. Semi-permanent colour is reasonably cheap and it is relatively easy to achieve good results in the salon or at home. Touches won't be necessary because a new application has to be repeated after four weeks or so.

Permanent Colour

This is usually a blend of a tint and hydrogen peroxide which penetrates the cortex and then is sealed in. The tint combines with your natural hair colour to produce the final shade.

○ Going a few shades *lighter* seems to work better than going *darker*, which can look flat and matte.

○ In a salon, tell them the history of your hair as it may affect how the tint takes; the initial treatment is always more expensive than later retouching treatments, so it is important to get it right.

○ At home, don't attempt to use a tint on previously bleached hair in the hope of improving the colour-it will probably end up looking brassy.

○ After tinting, be sure to condition your hair regularly.

60

- Tinting will normally need retouching every month or so, depending on how different it is from your natural colour.
- Permanent colour needs to grow out or be re-coloured by an expert.

Bleaching

Bleach tends to be ammonia-based (though there are ammonia-free varieties), mixed with hydrogen peroxide. It removes the natural pigment; a blonde toner then gives it the characteristic colour.

- Bleaching damages the hair so badly that it's best to resort to it only if you can't achieve blonde with a few shades of tint.
- It is expensive and time-consuming to return to your natural colour if you find that you don't like your hair bleached blonde.
- Salon bleaching always looks better than home-bleached hair.
- Your hair will need retouching, which not only means frequent visits to the salon, but each reapplication of bleach damages your hair further.

The New Generation

There are colourants that you can use at home or have applied in a salon, which are longer lasting than semi-permanents (which last for around 6 washes) but do not require the long-term commitment of a permanent colour. They last for 6-8 weeks, but don't lighten or damage the hair. In fact, these colourants will enhance the shine factor. Available in subtle and stronger shades, they are very effective at blending in grey hair.

Highlighting or Streaks

These are done by using a peroxide or tint mix that penetrates the hair cortex, applied by either the foil or cap method. Foil is usually more expensive but gives better results; pulling strands through a perforated rubber cap is a cheaper option.

Hair Colouring with Chemical Dye

This is meant for those who desire a permanent colouring of their hair in the desired shade. This readily available pack contains two bottles in the pack, one containing hydrogen peroxide (H_2O_2) and the other colouring material. Hydrogen peroxide is called developer which helps the colour penetrate deeply into the core of each hair to give long lasting colour to your hair (six to eight weeks). You can even lighten your hair. Most are shampooed on. Although the colour doesn't wash out, after every four weeks the roots will need re-touching. Modern applicators make it easy to apply the colour just where you want on the roots where the new hair growth is showing.

However, there is one great disadvantage that chemical dye makes the hair dry and porous, so you must use plenty of conditioners. The hair colourant now available in the market are also ammonia free. Ammonia is a strong alkali used to make the colour compound penetrate deeply. But the colourant formulated without it are less likely to irritate the skin. 'They don't smell as strongly either and leave hair in the better condition. Now permanent hair colouring products are available in two kinds : penetrating tints and coating tints—like the herbal hair dyes.

In fact initially you must go for professional help to camouflage grey hair. Tiny thread-like sections of hair are tinted all over the head, and as hair is made up of several different shades. The end results will show your hair in natural colour to a great extent.

Home-made Dyes : In all these dyes henna is the main colouring ingredient. Different shades are made by mixing Henna powders with water and lime juice. Take about 2 cupful of Henna powder, 1 cupful of warm water, 1 teaspoonful lime juice and stir the mixture vigorously to make a thick paste. Lime juice is mixed to make the dye release itself and give a uniform colour. Keep the paste aside for about one hour. Then apply it over your hair thickly and evenly. In case you desire darker shade mix one or two tablespoons of ground cloves. If you want to have dark brown shade mix one part of henna with 3 parts of indigo. A tablespoonful of coffee and 2 tablespoonful of 'Amla' powder mixed with henna also darken the shade to a desired degree.

Sometimes these dye might dry your scalp to an unpleasant degree in that case add a little of fresh curd (2 tbls.) and a small teaspoonful of mustard oil or 'sarson ka' oil. Wash the paste off your hair after about a couple of hours with a mild shampoo.

Another kind of home-made dye is that which is prepared with walnut shells. This is also a harmless dye which progressively adds colour to the hair. Part walnut shells in a mortar and cover with water. Add a touch of table salt and let it stand for 3 days. Now add three cups of boiling water and simmer for 5 hours, always ensuring that the evaporated water is religiously replaced. Now extract the dark liquid from the shells by means of press or by twisting the shells in a cloth. Replace separated liquid in the pot again and reduce to a quarter of its volume through boiling. Add a small piece of alum as fixative. At first it would produce a somewhat yellowish effect, but will finally give the hair a good deep black colour. Remember to use this dye on shampooed and clean hair.

Another kind of dye is made the following way : Take about a quart of water and add 4 teaspoons of any tea. Boil it until a very dark brown liquid is obtained. Alum is used to set the dye. Strain and use like a rinse. Repeat rinses until the desired shade is obtained. This concoction is believed to be even otherwise effective to fight the dandruff enhance. You can use this as rinse following dyeing your hair by home-made dyes.

On Choosing the Bright Shade for Your Hair.

Now since you are ready with your dyes of various kinds, what you should address yourself to is which shade would suit your hair best. Well, dye or no dye you cannot have your hair dyed in the natural colour as it looked when you were 25. The shade of the colour must match your existing complexion. If you have sallow or darker complexion browning your hair might look rather incontiguous. The general principle normally adhered to is : darker the hair the younger you should be. Jet-blacking your hair at 45 might make you look unnatural. You have to suit your hair-colour depending on your age.

Frequency of Dyeing Your Hair : The golden rule is to avoid overlapping of colour by retouching surfaces every week. If dyeing or bleaching is scheduled sooner you overprocess the previously treated hair. No matter what you do this is quite noticeable from the hair's dry and brittle appearance. If you colour of bleach five or six weeks later, you underlap the previously treated hair and eventually end up hair uneven structure of your hair. This is besides being running counter to the aesthetical requirement of your face is also harmful since the original chemical process of dyeing or bleaching alters the structure of the hair to begin with. Hence retouching after every four weeks is rather indispensable if you want your hair to look natural.

Also, there are some ladies who tend to put oil in their hair the day they dye it. This should never be done since you must allow your hair to remain dry at least for 72 hours to lit the process of oxidation complete.

Precautions in Dyeing Your Hair

(i) No matter which type of the dye you use to colour your hair always do the patch test, particularly so if you are using the market product. How to go about it is always mentioned in the precaution slip accompanying the dye. In case you detect any adverse reaction, take an antihistamine like. Avil and drink plenty of liquids to dilute the allergic effect besides washing off the experimental spot behind your left ear. Always be careful and never alter your dye brand frequently as this might even encourage the hair loss.

(ii) Now this point is very important. Normally people dye their hair after shampooing and making it clean. This is wrong. You must always use hair colour or bleach on hair in its soiled state. It is a mistake to shampoo it first, contrary to directions on most do-it-yourself products. It must be understood that the oil in hair actually protects the stain against the unwanted invasion of chemicals into the system. As a matter of fact on your 'dye-day' you shouldn't even brush your hair that morning.

(iii) Generally those who start dyeing the hair make the mistake of trying to eliminate any red pigmentation. But realise that red pigmentation is an important factor in the actual structure of the hair. If you try to remove the last link that holds the chain reaction of the hair itself together. Moreover when you darken your hair the red pigmentation highlights good aesthetically making it look most natural and charming. This is actually your asset and not a liability.

(iv) Sometimes the chemical effect of the market dyes show their adverse effect later on in reducing your heading power. In case you find even a slight change in your audio faculty, stop the use at once and consult a doctor.

(v) Highlighting is kinder than total bleaching; although it still damages your hair (sometimes leading it to knot easily and become frizzy), it *can* look wonderful, like naturally sun-streaked hair, giving the of depth and movement.

(vi) Bleaching is a technique best left to the salon, as there is too much room for mistakes with home kits.

(vii) On average, highlights will need to be redone every three months or so, though more frequent retouching may be necessary.

Vegetable Colours

These are colourants that use natural ingredients such as camomile or henna, the

(i) They add colour, depth and shine.

(ii) They are fairly cheap.

(iii) They can be used both at home and in the salon, although they tend not to work on grey hair unless they are specially designed for it, and highlighted and bleached hair may go a little orange.

(iv) The colour fades out gradually.

Colour Care

(i) Don't expose coloured hair to the sun as it will probably change its shade. Wear a hat or specialised hair protector.

(ii) Use shampoos produced specially for coloured hair.

❑

7

Shape and Style of the Hair

There is no hard and fast rule about shaping and styling of your hair. If all boils down to the fundamental requirement : that the style must add charms to your face. But while selecting your hair style, there are few principles that ought to be adhered to. The style must match your face and highlight its salient and attractive features. Hair designers are often asked questions about shapes and their proportions to hair styling. Keeping in mind the relationship to body height and styles you must strive to make your hair rather oval which is the ultimate in athletics.

The general strategy is to add height and fullness to areas that fall short. Closeness is imported when the area is extended. This way a balanced look is achieved. In any case it is important to increase or decrease the right amount of hair needed to create the proper hair-face relationship.

Remember that your hair style must appear in tandem with the body characterstics. Keep in mind that the normal proportion of head size to total height is measured at seven and half heads to height. Whatever the fashion mode of the day, hair should reflect its proper proportion in relationship to the body. In this regard you must give due weightage to the density, texture, weight and colour of the hair and the room for their natural variation.

Moreover, the new generation of styling aids have revolutionised hair-care and styling. Now we can inject life into our hair by building body, boosting, shine and fixing styles in just a few minutes since the modern age is 'Instant Age' and you have very little time for everything. Everything has to be accomplished quick and fast. Given below are some accessories that are needed to style your hair and give them the right (or desired) look.

Mousse

This is a fabulous, instant volume builder. It coats the hair making it easier to control and is especially useful for taming frizzy hair and for shaping the curl in permed hair. It will give energy to fine hair and extra texture to straight hair. Many mousses contain conditioners, which are excellent for dry ends.

Apply mousse by squeezing a golfball-sized knob of foam into the palm of your hand and then applying it with your fingers to the roots. Mousse is best applied to slightly damp hair because it will distribute better. Don't be tempted to use too much or you will overload the hair, and be careful to use very little on fine hair or you could end up with a sticky, heavy result.

Experiment with different strengths of mousse. It is often best to buy a mousse with a high hold factor and use less of it than to apply more of a lighter mousse.

If your hair feels lank later in the lay, spraying with a little water will revive it. Shape your hair with your fingers as it dries.

Gels

Gel defines texture on curly hair and will sleek and hold straight hair in place. There are several ways to use it. Gel can be applied to wet hair, combed into shape and then left to set hard. Or you can blow-dry the gelled hair, which gives lots of body and bounce but still leaves it looking silky and natural. Gel spreads more easily when applied to wet or slightly damp hair.

Gels, formulated for use on dry hair, are good for controlling small areas of hair and for slicking it back at the sides of your face. If the brand you are using becomes flaky, switch to another formulation.

. You can combine products such as mousses and gels or mousses and hairspray for extra styling strength.

Styling Lotions for Blow-drying

These spray-in lotions protect hair from the drying effects of heat when it is blow-dried. They also help to keep the hair cuticle flat, which prevents flyaway ends and increases shine. Many formulations will also help to increase volume.

Sculpting Lotions

These ultra-strong hair shapers are designed to be applied either to damp hair, which is then blowdried into shape, or to dry hair for fullness or uplifting effects.

Hairspray

You can use hairspray for localized styling and to keep your hair sleek. Hairspray holds a polished finish, but allows movement (which sculpting lotions do not). If you simply want to control a few stray ends, spray a little hairspray on to your brush and sweep it through your hair.

Hairspray is indispensable when the atmosphere is humid because it prevents the dampness from making your hair limp. Keep a mini hairspray in your bag-many pump sprays are reflillable.

Pomade and Wax

These are useful for thick hair, but should not be used on fine hair. Apply a little, using your fingertips to separate and define the hair—for instance, on a spiky fringe. Pomade and wax are terrific for creating shine and for controlling afro hair. Remember that they need to be washed out very thoroughly.

Serums

Fairly new on the market, serums are silicon-based liquids that tame frizzy ends, sleek flyaway hair and enhance shine on all hair types in seconds. You simply need a few drops, smoothed in the palm of your hands, then applied wherever you want. Good ones don't feel sticky.

Twist, Plaits and Rolls

As they say, modern classicism is today's way with hair looks. Hence there are multitude of stylish way to dress mid-length and long hair. We choose accessories according to our needs. As mentioned earlier we should consider our hair in terms of an overall look.

The beauty of mid-length and long hair is that it can be styled in an exciting variety of ways. Twists, plaits, braids, rolls and chignons all look super-stylish and can be worn with simple accessories to secure them in place, or decorated.

The key to success when styling is to apply a little mousse or gel to control flyaway ends and to sleek your hair before you start. You need to have a selection of long hairpins, kirby grips and covered elastics.

Twists

Quick to do, twists can be left soft and natural-looking— there is no need to plaster on hairspray!

Simply twist your hair along the side of your head on one side and fasten it at the back with a hair-clip.

Now twist back the other side and clip the two pieces together so that the hair hangs sleek and straight behind, or interweave the two twists at the nape of the neck and fasten with long hairpins.

Twists look pretty when several tortoiseshell chignon pins are placed around the twist.

Combs can be used to help hold twists in place. Look for combs without rough edges. Place them in your hair so that they grip by pushing the teeth up towards the crown of the head, then turn the comb and push it down.

Plaits, Braids, Rolls, French Pleats and Chignons

Plaits and Braids : Ideally you need to have hair of one length to plait and braid it quickly. Practice makes perfect plaits.

Braids (French plaits) are more tricky to do. Starting just below the crown of your head, divide the centre of your hair into three sections, plait these together and then pick up another section on either side of the centre piece and plait together again. Continue down to the nape of your neck and then plait as usual, fastening with a slide or covered elastic at the end.

Sharp, stylish and with a touch of formality, rolls are fun to wear with clothes that echo the style of the 1940s and 50s.

For a French pleat, take your hair back into the nape of the neck, twisting along the length of the hair. Roll the twist of hair upwards, turning the ends in, and fasten the pleat in place with pins.

These are good on fine to medium textured hair but take a little more time on heavier hair.

A low chignon placed at the nape of the neck looks modern. You can twist the hair and knot it, pulling the ends through the knot and securing with pins. Alternatively, you can take the hair into a low pony-tail, secure it with a covered elastic and then twist and pin into place.

Look out for hanky knots. These are especially shaped pieces of fabrics (raw silk ones look particularly good) which have an elasticated piece at one end. Simply place the fabric over the chignon and twist the elastic around twice to recure it.

The Guidelines to Select Your Hairstyle

Given below are some of the characteristic faces with their salient features to help you choose your style.

    (i) **Triangular Face :** This usually displays a jaw line that is somewhat incisive. In or to balance and detract, widen silhouette in symmetrical (balanced) form, and ease more hair on to the face to offset the irregularity and make the face more squarish.

(ii) **Square Face :** To a squarish face or the face whose jaw line is squarish, the effort should be to add height in the centre to minimise the squarishness. Adding slight width to further narrow the jaw would further obscure the square silhouette in the upper part.

(iii) **Long Face :** The facial structure should be dealt along the length to lessen the asymmetrical look. Don't add height but do increase some hair on the forehead to help giving a more ovalish look.

(iv) **Round Face :** This is better draft with improving the hair on face and by breaking the round hairline growth. Here the hair must appear to crowd the face horizontally. The hair should better be braided in the centre to give a longish look.

(v) With chin and forehead receding type, fullness over the forehead creates balance with the noseline and obscures the prominent shape.

(vi) With long jaw line face, the style should be such as balancing with proper positioning of the hair. Lowering of the side-hair motions on the face decrease the facial area in view.

(vii) If you have very low or small forehead, the hair should be styled in such a way that it creates the impression of height in the middle. A short hair-cut in front will give the forehead a higher look.

(viii) If you have long and sticking-out ear you should try to hide their prominence by adding more hair sidewards. The golden principle in hair styling is that you should attempt to make your face look as much oval as possible.

CHARMING HAIR STYLES

Sometimes it may puzzle you that, which hair-style would suit you for a special occasion or function, specially when you have little option. No problem, here we offer many hair-styles, you can choose easily.

If you have a long face and you want to hide it, choose this hair style. Here hair is cut from shoulders. On frontside they are cut just above the eyebrows giving a little uneven shape, so that it looks natural.

To give a gentle and innocent look, divide your hair into two equal parts, plait them behind your ears; then tie with rubber bands and pin them. Leave rest of the hair on your front.

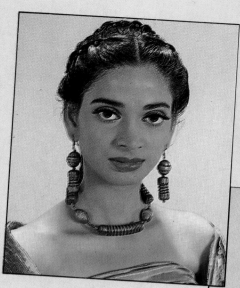

Divide your hair from centre and make plaits, tie pony. After dividing the pony into three parts, make plaits (choties) and tie them.

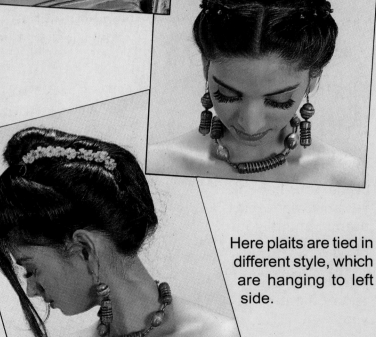

Here plaits are tied in different style, which are hanging to left side.

In this hair style, plaits are decorated diffrently.

This is French-roll. Here all the hair is taken on one side and have been pinned, then they are tied in a large bun.

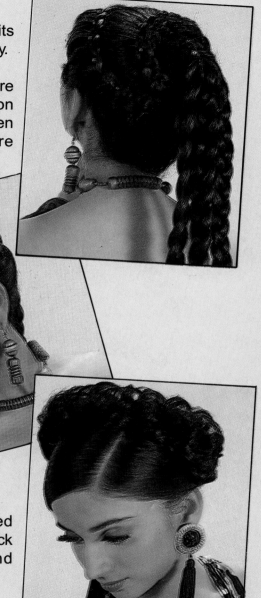

Here hair is divided from left side and back hair is curled and pinned beautifully.

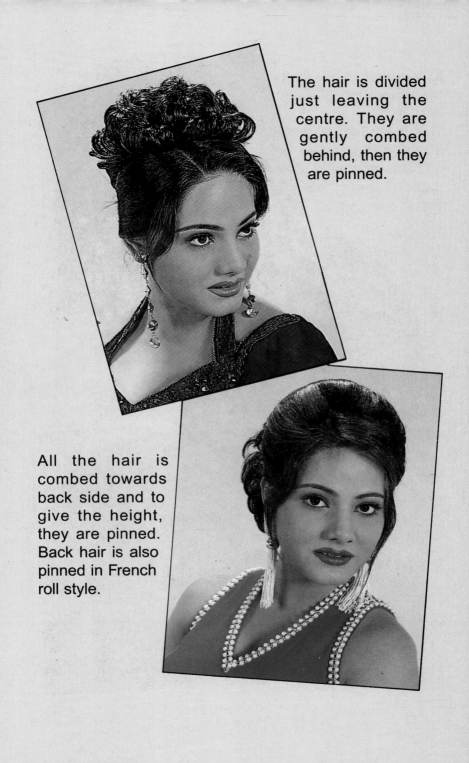

The hair is divided just leaving the centre. They are gently combed behind, then they are pinned.

All the hair is combed towards back side and to give the height, they are pinned. Back hair is also pinned in French roll style.

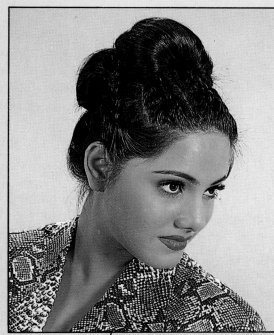

Here the front hair is divided into five parts and they are plaited and pinned on top. And on the back side, hair is tied in pony and four rolls are made from them.

The front hair has been divided into five parts and plaited in different style.

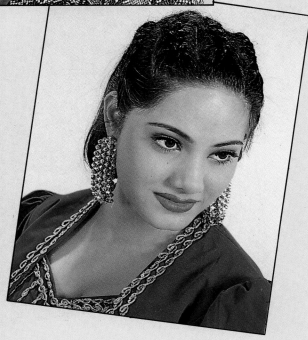

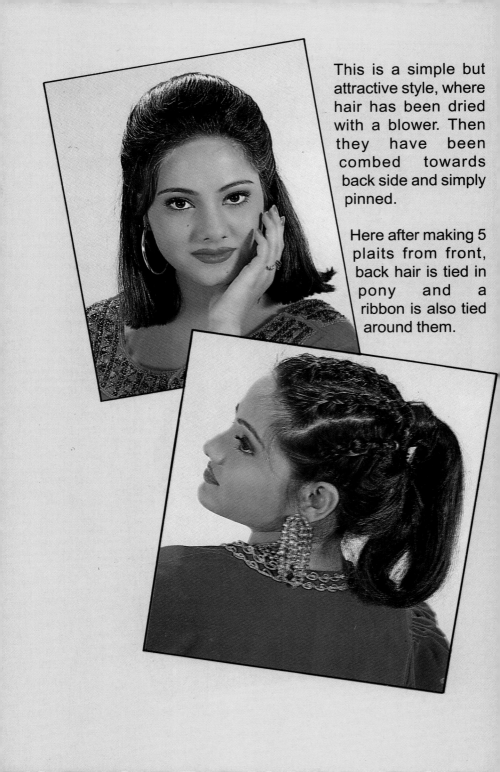

This is a simple but attractive style, where hair has been dried with a blower. Then they have been combed towards back side and simply pinned.

Here after making 5 plaits from front, back hair is tied in pony and a ribbon is also tied around them.

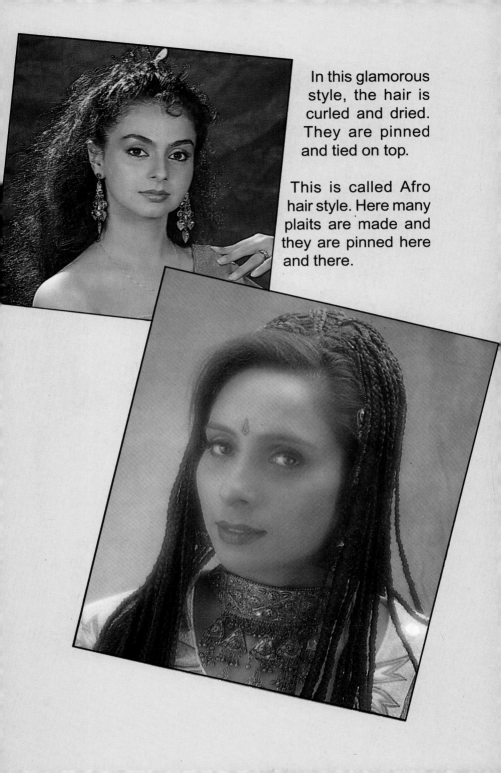

In this glamorous
style, the hair is
curled and dried.
They are pinned
and tied on top.

This is called Afro
hair style. Here many
plaits are made and
they are pinned here
and there.

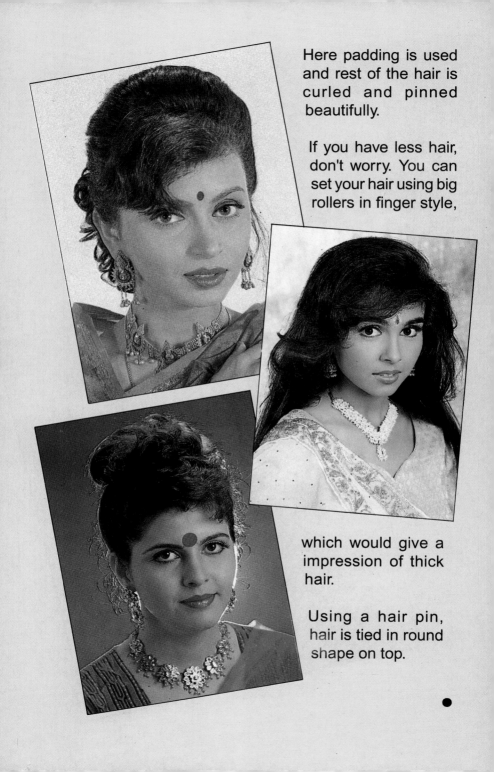

Here padding is used and rest of the hair is curled and pinned beautifully.

If you have less hair, don't worry. You can set your hair using big rollers in finger style,

which would give a impression of thick hair.

Using a hair pin, hair is tied in round shape on top.

8

Clever Hair Cutting Techniques

Many Indian women don't realise that a good haircut is the basis of a great hairstyle and will keep your hair in top condition.

Your hairstyle can make all the difference to whether you feel confident and happy with your appearance or dissatisfied. It is important therefore to find a hairdresser with whom you can develop a good rapport.

A stylist will adapt a cut according to your hair type and the directions of hair growth, and ensure that the style will enhance your features and flatten the shape of your face. He or she should also take your lifestyle into account and give you a cut that's easy to maintain. Do take with you photographs of styles you like, but be prepared to be flexible if the hairdresser feels they won't work on your hair type. Equally, try to be open to new ideas, as changing your hairstyle is the most effective way to inject new energy into your look.

Regular Cuts

You should have your hair cut approximately every 6-8 weeks, although a very precise short style may need shaping every 4 weeks.

Changing Your Hairdresser

If you're thinking about changing stylists, book a free consultation or a simple service such as a trim before opting for a major new look. This will give you a chance to find out if you're on the same wavelength!

SHORT CUTS

Short hair can be cut and styled to create many different looks, from the classic short bob to the gamine urchin image. Sharp, angular styles look strong and individual; then there are soft, wavy styles that are modern classics. The added bonus with short hair is that it can look professional and smart in an instant.

Versatile Bobs

The classic short bob remains modern-looking and is easy to style and wear. Blunt cut on straight hair the bob looks chic and shiny. A short bob just below the ears looks young and fun.

Layering a bob gives the effect of movement. A layered bob can be worn full and wide, scrunch-dried and teased out with the aid of mousse, or close to the face, with the sides swept forwards. A permed bob with a straight fringe is a variation on the theme.

Your hairdresser will advise you as to whether a side parting or a fringe is best for you. Asymmetric cuts work well on the bob shape and add an element of individuality.

The Urchin Look

Gamine cuts that are short, layered and cut close to the head look especially chic when worn slightly tousled.

MID-LENGTH AND LONG HAIR

Whether one-length and sleek, or layered and full, longer hair can make you feel especially glamorous. It is, however, essential to keep longer hair in peak condition—keep brushing to a minimum and do it gently. Have it trimmed regularly, too, so that split ends don't have a chance to develop—they'll simply work their way up the hair shaft.

Volume with Length

If you want to wear your hair long but like height on top, you could try a 'no curl' perm just on the roots. Alternatively, for temporary lift, use large velcro rollers. Roll sections of hair under, spritz with setting lotion or hairspray and then brush out.

Fringe appeal

Consider keeping interest at the front if your hair is long. A fringe can be short and straight, or longer and layered.

Pre-Raphaelite Curls

Curls can be created with curling tongs or by sleeping with your hair in rags. Twist a lock of hair and wind it round your finger. Insert the end of a strip of fabric through the hole created by your finger and fasten it with a knot. Long-lasting curls can be achieved with a spiral perm.

Care for Long Hair

Long hair is believed to be an ultimate symbol of modernity at least in India. Shining long hair, flowing loose or carefully dressed adds grace to a female personality that no hair style can. Even in this age of change and controversy it is still believed that beauty and the inevitable sex appeal.

Of course, long hair does add charm to the personality but one has to pay price for it. It is because when long hair isn't properly cared for, it begins to look like a rough rope made of straw.

Hence what is most needed is keeping the hair neat and clean by regularly shampooing it with the shampoo found most suitable. Also since hair is long, the wet bunch of hair need all the more care since wetness make the hair more fragile and breakable.

Following shampoo-wash, don't brush your hair instantly wrap it in a towel to blot out some of the moisture. Rubbing splits the hair-ends and tugging very wet hair in its weakened state, pulls out the hair. It is only when your hair is slightly dry-that you should comb it with a wide-loothed comb, starting from the ends slowly working up to the crown. This is how you can easily avoid tangles and excessive pressure on the hair roots.

Some times many ladies face a queer problem : oily scalp coupled with dry and split-ends. Follow your shampoo with a final rinse of diluted vinegar. Put just one tablespoon of vinegar to a mugful of water. For restoring the acid mantle of the scalp that has been just washed. It ought to be followed by creamy conditioner only at the ends. Oily hair also requires brushing to keep oil from pooling on the scalp and to carry the oil to hair ends to prevent the ends from drying out and eventually splitting into twain.

The long-hair care needs one very important tool : Correct brush with correct method of brushing your hair. Recommended is a brush with natural bristles or rounded synthetic bristles set in a back that is durable with a handle which fits comfortably in your hands. The best way to brush your hair is with your head hung down, while you brush finely from nape to ends of hair and all round. Use firm, even strokes. Also, don't tear your hair and don't yank it.

Frequent massage of the scalp is also recommended by leading trichologist. There is no doubt that massage of the scalp loosens the scalp and improves the circulation, giving elasticity to the hair. Start massaging with the fingers together at the top of your hair using cushions and not the fingertips. Use rotatory motion to massage your hair with the cushions while occasionally using the fingertips to reach the areas not easily reachable by the cushions.

In case of the long hair rough treatment invariably given rise to the problem of split hair since fierce brushing snaps the hair and breaks it off. There are certain appertenances used in styling your hair cause problem with the long hair. Like the use of rubber bands to tie hair together and winding hair into a fish

84

look with metal curbers and rollers. What you should do for avoiding split-ends is to treat your hair gently. First trim the hair gently about some distance from the split-end. Keep them under control by using a cream conditioner on the dry ends. Those with long hair should avoid using metal or wire rollers.

It has been generally noticed that the girls who wear long hair in tight plaits and women who wear a tight chignon seems to be the most frequent victims of spot baldness. It is invariably caused by pulling the hair tightly back in an elastic band or hum in exactly the same place for a long period. The position of a ponytail or a hum and the parting of these hair-do showed be changed often if loss of hair is to be avoided-some of the treatments given for checking spot-boldness in the earlier pages may also be taken recourse to. Hair pulled back into confined styles should have the benefit of extra care in correct brushing and massage.

The ladies or girls with long hair should sparingly use the electric rollers, curling irons and blow-driers and be sure to condition their hair after shampoo and use hot oil treatments to stop your hair getting dry and eventually develop split ends problem.

The Choice of Length of Hair

Of course it is totally according to your convenience and, possibly the requirement of the face cut and body frame but we prefer to advise you as to how you should trim them so that your choice is fulfilled.

(i) **Straight Cut :** This cut trims the strands exactly round the neck although this length can be extended upto waist. This cut suits best for a round face, seems to elongate your face a bit. Those with long hair shouldn't go for this cut and also those with thin hair.

(ii) **U-Cut :** This cut trims the hair in such a wave as to make the end form a parabolic shape heading downwards, the longest strand just below the neck and the line usually rise up proportionately from both the ends.

(iii) **Shag Cut :** Ideally suited for dense and curly hair with long stature and broad face. But in the case the parting must be not in the middle. With ladies or girls of this cut of hair not the sari but maxie that would be suiting most.

(iv) **Boy Cut :** As the name suggests this is what the boys generally go for. Meant especially for the 'mod' with jeans and top, although even with sari this might look good on some with an intellectual look.

(v) **Shoulder Cut :** When trimming is done almost at the shoulder level. It is better to have your hair rolled at the end of their length.

(vi) **Bob-Cut :** This suits more the young girls rather than mature ladies, with broad face, slim neck (but with a look of fulness). In this 'bob cut' too the parting should be not in the middle.

(vii) **Six Steps :** In case you are interested in keeping your hair untied, this cut would be ideal for you. In this case the hair is cut at three level. First, cut at close to eye-brow level; second, around the ears and the last cut in bottom-level in U-shape. Parting again should be shifted to one side.

❑

9

Permanent Solutions

This technique sets your hair as you desire, almost permanently. Whether you want cascading curls or little extra volume, a perm will inflect vitality into your hairstyle. In short they are termed as perming solutions or only perming.

Modern perms are incredibly versatile. You can have your hair permed for volume, to give bounce, curls or ringlets, for root movement (which is good for limp hair) and to give support to a style without any curl at all. They work on almost any length of hair, too.

Perming Process

Perming alters the hair's chemical bonds so that new links are forged around the curler. After the perm has taken, the perming solution is rinsed out with water and the curls are then locked into place with a neutralising lotion.

The softness of the perm depends on the size of the perming rod that is used. Large curlers produce softer perms, while small curlers give tight perms. Varying sizes and shapes of perming rods can be used, according to your hair type and the effect

87

required. The hair can also be rolled in different directions to achieve different styles.

Pre-perm tips

A skin allergy test and test curl are advisable if you are new to perming or if your hair is in bad condition. As perming is a complicated technical process, it is wise to have it done professionally.

Hairdressers frequently use a deep-cleansing treatment before perming in order to remove residues from conditioners and styling products from the hair.

Perm Types

'Acid' and 'alkaline' perms are available. 'Alkaline' perms are more successful, in general, on virgin hair as it is stronger than 'acid' perming lotion. Hair itself is acid-based, so 'acid' perms are considered safer for coloured and highlighted hair. Both types of perm can last the same length of time—there is no set lifespan for a perm, it depends on how quickly your hair grows.

Some perms claim to restructure the hair, restoring up to 90 per cent of its original strength, and to provide on-going conditioning.

Keratin, the protein found in hair itself, and natural moisturising factors are locked into the hair cortex and so act as a system of 'molecular mending'.

Post-perm Tips

- O Once a perm has been neutralised properly it is fixed, so there is no need to avoid shampooing it for 24 hours.
- O Avoid two-in-one shampoo and conditioner which can be too heavy.
- O Have your hair trimmed every 6 weeks, as extra weight will pull the curl down.
- O Curl reactivators are effective for restoring bounce.
- O Avoid brushing permed hair as this will create static

and separate the curls. Use a wide-toothed comb instead.

○ Where a perm is too curly you can try setting it on large rollers, or gently blow-dry the curl out using a big round brush.

The Frequency of Perming : As the name implies, curl is permanently waved in the hair. Although the curl may relax a little after shampooing and day to day wear, it will never entirely go away. But as the hair grows and you have the hair cut, your perm may be cut off. The new growth from the scalp will be again straight and hence the next session of perming may be required after about every three to four months. You may judge it yourself as to when your desired perm is losing its shape and style and body. There is no hard and fast rule about it and you can repeat perming operations when you feel you need them.

Where to Go for Perms ?

Since perming solutions contain some chemicals which might not be entirely in agreement with your scalp and hair, their little under or overuse is not likely to give the desired results apart from the excessive use of the solutions proving damaging your hair. At times the home perming results in under processing— meaning there may be no desired curl or perm. In contrast to this hazard your hair-stylist, with his or her professional knowledge would know exactly which strength of perm solution, rod size and wrapping technique is best suited to your hair and its style recommended for. The hair stylist must be knowing about the time factor which is very vital far perming. Moreover, in today's busy schedules when most women are working to support their family's sustenance in they may not get much time for their own hair perming. A professional hand would need one-and-half to two-and-half hours for the service, the major part of which is generally the wrapping of the hair on the perm rods. You must be prepared for spending this much time when you visit a salon. This should never be a rush job since time is a vital factor in good perming.

As far as the cost factor is concerned, like normal hair cutting price depends upon the salon, grade of professional service, stylist, condition of your hair, so does perming. But few hundreds you must shell out to have an important fashion accessory. After all, all the twenty four hours you must wear it and even more.

Should you go for perming before or after your hair cut ? This too depends on your stylist, your personal style performance and the condition of your hair. For this you must seek your professional stylist's advice.

You can go perming even if you have curly hair for redirecting the natural curl into a more manageable pattern or to achieve a particular look or style. In case you wish to convert small curls into larger curls, go for perming on larger rods for achieving the desired results.

Some Guidelines for Perming

(i) In case you have skin abrasiveness or scalp irritation, it is advisable to tell your stylist and wait till these conditions are cured or at least made better. Because some solutions and lotions used in perming make aggravate these conditions.

(ii) Also, some medications do build up on the hair shaft and they can surely interfere with the perming results.

(iii) In many cases, some people misuse there hair rather quite callously. First of all they need to have their hair medically treated before they go for perm service.

(iv) Because of the above-mentioned precautions it is always better to go for perming when you have consulted your trichologist.

❑

10

General Instructions For Good Hair-Care

Although through different chapters we have tried to cover the entire range of the hair-care, this chapter is devoted to the essentials mentioned in each chapter and analysing the basic requirements as an organic whole. The basic requirements are the following :

(i) **Shampoo :** A shampoo is an indispensable first requirement for good maintenance of your hairy crown. Of course the age-old principle is struck to one brand but you don't know what you might be using is not the ideal choices for your hair. It is better to select at least two to three shampoos and stick to your choice depending upon the vagaries of weather. For what may be good for the winters might not be good for the rainy season. Also, summers might require yet another kind of shampoo.

Remember that depending upon the external conditions the best shampoo is that which keeps the PH level of your scalp normal and which has enchanting scent. Ask friends or your hair-dresser for recommendations.

91

Once you have selected your ideal shampoo or a set of shampoos to cope with the vagaries of weather, you must decide the frequency of its use. It mainly depends upon your occupation or nature of work. If you are a housewife you might not require to shampoo your hair frequently. Those who go out to work may require to shampoo their hair more frequently. Remember that no matter how good the cut or how pretty the style, your hair can't look its best if it isn't clean, fluffy and manageable. In case you are required to shampoo frequently you should go for a simple hairstyle.

(ii) **Conditioner :** A good shampoo might require an occasional hair conditioning, which requires a good hair conditioner. Hair that is washed frequently, permed or coloured, or regularly exposed to heated hair appliances surely needs a hair conditioner. Although your hair-dresser, again may be the best one to advise you, yet generally choose an instant liquid conditioner to apply after each shampoo. Once a month treat your hair and scalp to a deep conditioning treatment for extra nourishment. If your hair is damaged, use the deep conditioner more often, say, two or three times a month. Also remember that a damaged hair can't be repaired by any hair conditioner. A hair conditioner cannot cure it, only makes it look and feel better. In case your hair is damaged cut off the damaged part before starting your conditioning operations.

(ii) **Blow-Drier :** It is generally held that repeated exposure of hair to blowers-cum-drier of all sizes and wattage damages the strands you will have to select the size, range etc. of these accessories but also their frequency of operation over your head. See which of them you find most useful apart from their being handy. Those with travelling job should go for those blow-driers that are easily packed.

(iv) **Curling Iron :** Of course using them for creating desired curls is not feasible for working persons but it is great for brief touch-ups and quick curls. It is also available in portable varieties, ideal for reviving a withered or wilted hairstyle.

(v) **Combs and Brushes :** We have repeatedly been touching upon their ideal quality but the truth is that you have to select them in accordance to your need, your hair-quality and their usefulness. Only precaution one must always take is ensuring that the nylon-brushes have their tips rounded. Any unrounded nylon bristle might cut straight across and damage your hair. The best combs—from the point of view of holding them and conveniently running them through hair—is that with a handle or 'tail'. As for the brushes, after you blow-dry your hair the ideal brush is that with a round natural brushes. These brushes come in many sizes. You choose the size according to your need—the larger brushes create fuller, loose style while the smaller ones are best for a tightier, curlier look.

(vi) **Tools and Accessories for Setting :** Rollers either the foam kind or hard plastic ones come handy if electric appliances don't do your hair job to your satisfaction. These rollers will give you a full and fluffy style. But it is advisable not to go in for brush rollers or rollers secured with hair picks as they both tend to break or damage your hair. There are also available bobby pins or chips that can be effectively used for producing curls right from fine nipples to deep waves.

Those who use the setting aids manage to save a lot of time you can put more hair on each roller if you take advantage of these setting aids and in that case your hairstyle will outlive the styles set by gels and lotions.

Plain barretles or small hair combs come handy to 'repair' a fallen hairstyle, In case you keep your hair long you can sweep it back with a coated band. Keep these in your bag to help you set your hair in a short notice.

What You Should Look In For Choosing Your Hairdresser

(i) The hairdresser should give you a style that fits both your hair type and your life-style. In case you spend a great deal of time outdoors on the job or off, you don't need a hair-style that needs constant protections from the vagaries of matter. The same is true in a damp and windy climate.

(ii) The hair-dresser should not only be an expert in his or her job, the person must have enough knowledge to encourage your learning a few vital tips yourself about trichology in the sense that you may be able to do your hair job yourself in case you are not able to visit the person on scheduled time. If you feel even the professional job needs retouching, your should change your hair-guide (the hairdresser).

(iii) Reputation in these sphere is best carried by word of mouth. Ask your friends, relations etc. to guide you to the good hairdresser. As they say the proof of pudding lies in its eating. So if you happen to see someone carrying a hairstyle you admire most, search for that hairdresser. It is for sure that a good hair dresser is as important in your hair-upkeep and maintenance as all shampoos and conditioners put together. Don't be daunted by the high charges. Remember if one survives in the market despite the charges being high, then that must be a good hairdresser.

❏

11

How to Get Rid of The Unwanted Hair ?

Many readers might object inclusion of this chapter in this book on 'Hair-Care'. But, is it not the fact that this chapter ought to have been included in every book on this subject. That kind of hair also grow on body and its removal is as important as caring for hair on head. Though people might not disclose they do get worried by this kind of hair, when they try to remove it they face many problems. It is with this consideration that we thought to devote a separate chapter on this topic.

Why must such hair grow ? It is the activity of the endocrine glands that escalates during puberty, menopause or due to certain internal disorders. The growth of superfluous hair accompanies the hormonal changes that occur. During puberty, hormonal disturbance is characterised with erratic menstrual cycle, under developed breasts and often hairiness. Psychologically the dark-haired ladies are often distressed with their excess hair problem, when they actually have no more than usual. It is pure visual fallacy caused by their dark hair that make them unnecessarily worried. The real problem is 'Hirsutism' and is considered hereditary to a large extent.

95

Also the hair growth is triggered off due to other hormonal imbalance caused by tumors, cysts of the ovaries, malfunctioning and tumors of the other endocrinal glands, such as the pituitary and thyroid.

It has also been noticed that stress and tension are negative factors in the excessive hair growth. The hair follicles are under the influence of hormones. Emotional stress and anxiety disturb the normal activity which stimulates the hair follicles on our body.

However, there are certain drugs that do adversely react and trigger off the symptoms of 'Hirstism' like 'hydrocortisone' and 'delandome' generally found in birth control pills, cosmetic creams etc. Hence these drugs must always be taken only when prescribed by a registered practitioner.

There are many methods of removing these superfluous hair. Some of them are given below. But since every method is not likely to suit everyone, it is advisable to employ them after a prior test.

   (i) **Electrolysis :** This is the permanent solution to removing unwanted hair, though hormonal changes during the life cycle can cause new hair growth. Other treatments are only temporary. (see ahead).

   (ii) **Depilatory Creams :** These creams dissolve the hair to just below the surface of the skin. The pain factor is zero in them unless you experience an allergy. It is important to do a patch test 24 hours beforehand. Depilation will be necessary again after a week or so.

       Although depilatory creams are quick and effective but fairly messy to use and often smell unpleasant.

   (iii) **Shaving :** Probably the most popular type used at home for hair removal. It cuts the hair down to the surface of the skin, removing some of the skin's outer layer.

       Pain factor is zero unless you cut yourself. It takes only a few minutes to complete the operation. As far as regrowth is concerned, the fact is that it starts to look and feel stubby after a couple of days. Hence it needs redoing at least twice a week to keep smooth. Hair also grows somewhat coarser than before. The coarseness of the hair also tends to blacken the area progressively.

Few Tips For Smooth Shaving

To prevent irritation, use moisturising shave cream and a razor with a comb guard.

Use a special electric shaver for the sensitive Irkini line.

If you are off to the beach, shave the day before to allow the skin to recover—soreness can be triggered by chlorine, sunscreens and perspiration.

(iv) **Waxing :** This can be done both at home and in the salon though salon waxing tends to be more effective.

Wax is usually heated and then pulled off in strips with paper or gauze against the direction of the hair growth, pulling hair out from the follicle. Most salons use the cold (in fact lukewarm) wax system. Hot waxing is less widely available and is less hygienic as the wax is filtered and reused.

You will feel a quick pain—Ouch! Stings, but it is over in a flash. You get used to it. Remember that your skin will be more sensitive before menstruation.

Time taken in waxing operation (both legs, knees to ankles) is about 10 minutes.

Regrowth is anything from three to six weeks. Hair grow back finer after repeated treatment.

In waxing hair has to be long enough to be covered by the wax. If it is too short, it either won't come out or will be removed patchily to the surface only, with disapproving results. Never employ this method on broken or irritated skin.

To minimise irritation the skin should be pulled taut before stripping. Afterwards little pimple may break out, but they generally subside after a few days. To avoid further irritation, for the next 24 hours avoid the sun, very hot showers, products containing alcohol or fragrance, deodorant if the underarms have been waxed and strenuous activity which might cause perspiration.

In case you find ingrowing hairs after waxing, use an exfoliator to help them grow in the right or desired direction.

Also remember that waxing has to be done regularly.

(iv) **Sugaring :** This is a new method called sugar-and-water putty, applied to the small area at a time and pulled off against the hair growth. It is well known in the Middle East and is becoming increasingly available in salons elsewhere.

It is marginally less painful than waxing. As far as time taken is concerned half-leg sugaring will take about 45 .minutes. It is done comparatively in more laid-back style than waxing and in the Arab countries it is most popular. Many people replace sugar with honey in the putty. Regrowth in this style of hair removal would take anything from four to six weeks but it generally depends upon the hair growth. Hair grows back slower and finer with successive treatment. Hence those who wish to remove the problem as little as possible in the hope of its altogether removal generally go for it.

Although sugaring has this advantage and is also less expensive than waxing yet there are not many salons which do this job. It is generally done at home and hence needing more time.

The after-waxing tips given above also apply in this case of sugaring as well.

(v) **Threading :** It is an ancient Chinese art that is very popular in India as well. The therapist winds a piece of thread round one forefinger, forms a loop with it and whisks the hair out. It hardly causes any pain, just a sting is felt. Time taken is dependent on the size of the area being treated. Fine hair may not regrow up to 12 weeks. The regrowth shall be much finer than the original hair (if a therapist is unskilled and cuts the hair off at the surface, it looks—thicker. Eventually the hair growth becomes weaker and can stop altogether.

Threading is best suited to facial hair and much preferred by therapists to wax on this delicate skin.

(vi) **Electrolysis (II) :** Although we have already mentioned about this process, this is being referred to again for some precautions. In this method hair should be treated during its growing cycle after 2-3 treatments. It is possible to time the sessions to remove the new growth.

Electrolysis involves inserting a needle (phase ensure that your salon uses disposable ones) into the follicle and destroying the hair with heat generated by an electric current.

The 'blend' method combines two currents and it is more popular as it can produce faster results.

Pain felt is like a short, sharp wince. It varies from surface to surface.

Time taken is from 5 minutes to half an hour depending on the area treated and your pain threshold. As hairs must be caught during an active cycle it can take months to eradicate hair completely.

Regrowth is very slow during this treatment. Once treatment is finished, it is almost negligible.

Electrolysis needs especial care not only from the expert's side but also from your side. You need to be dedicated to undergo this treatment. Of course it is most effective but it is a lengthy process.

It can become expensive, depending upon the area and strength of hair growth being treated. It is not, for example, economically viable to have your legs treated in this manner.

It should never be done at home lest you might sear yourself permanently. In the cases of black skins electrolysis can also produce areas of darker pigment.

Remember not to schedule your appointment just before a meeting or going out if you are having electrolysis on the face, as there will be a little puffiness and redness afterwards, although this goes after a few hours.

❑

12

Yoga and Hair-Care

Many might be surprised to read this chapter. But the following Asanas have been found particularly good for ensuring lush hair growth.

1. Sarvangasana
2. Sarpasana
3. Kukkutasana
4. Shuturmurghasana
5. Vajrasana
6. Chakrasana
7. Shavasana

In fact, all these Asanas restore the hormonal balance in the body and regulate the circulation of blood hence they have beneficial effect on the hair as well. We shall be discussing these Asanas one by one.

1. **Sarvangasana :** This literally means the (yogic) exercise for all organs of the body. Sarvangasana is made of three Sanskrit words: 'sarva' means all, 'anga' means organs and 'asana' means exercise or posture. By revitalising the whole body by energising thyroid and parathyroid glands it keeps the body and hence hair in 'most fit' condition.

Technique :

Stage (a) : Raising the legs. Place a folded blanket on the ground. Lie flat on your back with both legs straight and together.

100

Now straighten your arms and place them besides the body, palms downwards.

For a few seconds completely relax the whole body. During the next movement, raising the body, the breath can be retained inside or outside. That is you hold your breath. Now slowly raise your legs by contracting and utilising the abdominal muscles. The movement should be gradual with control, it should take at least 10 seconds for the legs to reach vertical position. Keep the legs straight and together. If possible try to raise the legs using only abdominal muscles for this action will help you straighten these muscles. At the end of the movements the buttocks should be back on the ground with the legs pointing directly upwards.

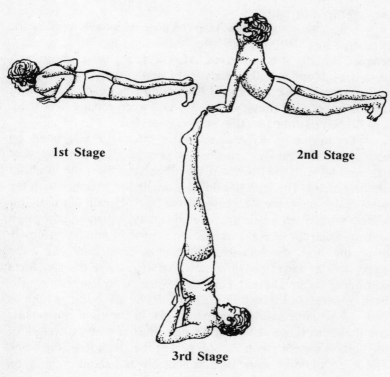

1st Stage

2nd Stage

3rd Stage

Stage (b) : Taking the final pose. In this stage the arms and hands should take an active part in assuming the final position. Elevate the legs further off the ground by pressing the hands and arms, the nape of the neck, back of the head and shoulders. Close the eyes. Try to relax the whole body. Breath deeply and slowly. Beaware of the breathing.

Stage (c) : Returning to the starting position. Stay in the finally reached position as long as you can. Then fold the straight legs over head so that the feet above and behind the back of the head. Slowly raise the position of the hands behind the chest and place the arms flat on the floor. Slowly lower the buttocks to the floor. Then gradually rotate the straight legs over the top of the head and lower them to the ground again while not using as much as possible the assistances of arms. Now completely relax the body when it is once again flat on the ground. Reach all the position mentioned above, slowly and rhythmically. There should be no jerky movement.

Who shouldn't do this Asana? Those who have weak heart, excessive high BP. Though after some time the BP is greatly reduced initially it is increased. Also pregnant ladies those who have weak blood vessels, excessively enlarged thyroid and those with a slipped disc history. This shouldn't be practised with in three hours of your filling your belly. Also when you are ill or tired.

2. Sarpasana (or the Snake Pose)

Technique : Lie flat on a blanket spread on the ground, on your stomach. Fold your arms behind your back clasping the wrist of one hand with the fingers of the other hand. Rest the forehead on the ground. The legs should be straight and together with the soles facing upwards. Relax the whole body. Breath normally for a short time. Then inhale deeply and slowly, expanding the chest and abdomen as much as possible. At the end of inhalation slowly bend the head backwards. When you have bent the head backwards as far as possible slowly start to raise the shoulders and upper back. The movement is executed by contracting the back muscles and thrusting the arms. Raise the body as high as you can without causing any strain. Hold the final pose while continuing to retain the breath inside. Ensure that the weight of the body is supported on the soft part of the abdomen—the belly. The legs should be as relaxed as possible and should remain on the floor throughout. After a comfortable length of time slowly lower the body to the floor while exhaling. Completely relax the body in the starting position. Allow respiration to return to normal. Then repeat the asana up to five times. All these stages are to be achieved gradually and in a piecemeal fashion.

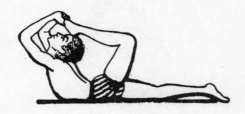

Difficult Variation

Inhale while in the starting position; this should be as deep as possible for this has much influence on the benefits obtained. Retain the body while raising the body and maintaining the final pose. Exhale while lowering the body to the ground again. Be always aware of breathing and movement. Stay in the final pose as long as you can retain your breath.

Those people who suffer from stomach ulcers, high blood pressure, heart troubles or hernia shouldn't do this exercise, as also the pregnant lady.

Its one difficult variation—provided you have strong back muscles—is interlocking the thumbs and holding the arms straight and on each side of the head, so that the lungs, trunk and arms lie in one straight line. Another variation is bringing the two legs over your head turn by turn and holding it with your both hands as shown below.

(3) **Kukkutasana :** A cock is called Kukkuta in Sanskrit, hence the name.

Technique : First sit in the posture of Padmasana. This is achieved the following way. While sitting on the ground, stretch

103

your legs forward. Keep them together. Place the right foot on the left thigh and the left foot on the right thigh in such a manner that the heels of both the feet touch the abdomen, on the sides of the navel. Keep the hands on the knees. Keep the body, back and head erect. The knees of both the feet should touch ground and generally the eyes should remain closed. One should do Pranayam also in this pose.

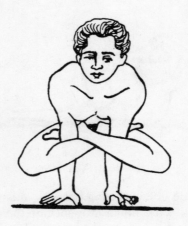

Kukkutasana

Now for Kukkutasana insert your hands between the opening in your calves and things. Then push the hands further and keep your palms firmly planted on the floor with your finger fully spread. Push your thighs and legs up your arms, using your arms exerting the force to lift your body up. Try to keep your torso as upright as possible breaths normally. Do it at least for a minute. The pregnant ladies shouldn't do it.

(4) **Shuturmurghasana :** For the hair another asana good is Shuturmurgasana. For this, keep your legs straight, bend from your waist and try to touch the toes or even the floor. This you can do with a little practice. Let your hair fall fully on to the floor (in case you keep them long). Hold it for a few seconds and then gradually assume your standing pose.

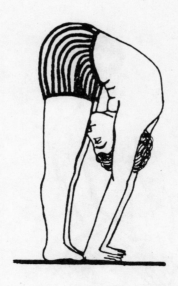

Shuturmurghasana

Important : Needless to emphasise that the pregnant ladies can't do either of these Asanas. But before and after pregnancy they must do it so that they keep their hair free from the various troubles. As our readers might have noticed all those Asanas are good for hair which either bring there hair down or head. It is the movement of the head coupled with exercises that activate the blood circulation that are generally found good for hair.

(5) **Vajrasana :** Vajra means thunderbolt in Sanskrit. Since this asana makes the body as strong as thunderbolt, it is so named.

Technique : Kneel down on the floor with your knees, ankles and big toes touching the ground. Now sit down on your heels and place your palms on the knees. Keep yourself erect but relaxed. Breath should be deep, even and slow. Now expand your chest and draw the abdominal region inwards.

This asana even the pregnant ladies up to the initial five months can also do. It removes the spinal problems and even tones up sexual organs of both male and female. You can do it even after having your meals.

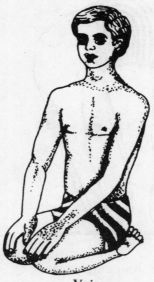

Vajrasana

(6) **Chakrasana :** Chakra in Sanskrit means a wheel, hence
the name.

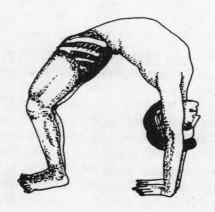

Chakrasana

106

Technique : Lie flat on your back. Bend the legs and place the heels near the buttocks, the feet should be about half a metre apart. Bend the arms and place the hands on the ground besides the back of the head; the fingers should point towards the shoulders with the palms flat on the floor.

Now relax the whole body for a few seconds in preparation for performing the final pose. Breath in deeply. Then raise the head and trunk off the ground straightening the legs and arms, the feet and hands should not be moved. Now try to arch back as much as possible to take the final pose.

Let the head hang between the two straight arms. The degree of bend in the neck can be accentuated by bending or straightening the knees and allowing the shoulders to move over the arms. Don't overstretch the back in arching it. This is the final pose. Breath slowly and deeply. Stay in the final pose for as long as it is comfortable. Then slowly return to the starting position by gradually lowering the body to the ground. This asana can be repeated once or twice if you have sufficient energy and time.

Chakrasana should not be practised by people who suffer from stomach ailments like ulcerative colitis, dilated eye pupils or hernia. In case you have recently undergone any abdominal operation, do not do it. Also, pregnant ladies shouldn't practise it at all.

(7) **Shavasana :** This asana is also known as mritasana. Shava means corpse, hence the name.

Technique : Lie flat on your back in the supine position. Place a small pillow on a folded blanket behind your head with the corners pulled under the shoulders. This ensures relaxation of your neck and shoulder muscles. Rest your arms in line with and on each side of your body. The palms should face upwards and the hands should not be clinched. The legs should be straight and slightly separated. Now close your eyes. Try to feel different parts of your body in contact with the floor. This is most important for it starts to develop your awareness of the different parts of the body. Feel the contact between the floor and the buttocks. Keep your attention on the pressure between the floor and the buttocks for a few seconds until you think that this area of the body is relaxed. Now try to feel the contact between the ground

107

and the right heel for a few seconds. Repeat the same thing with the left heel. Now feel the contact between the floor and the right arm, right hand, left arms, left hand, the middle of the back, each shoulder-blade in turn, the back of the body, the back of the head—in short each limb of your body separately. Try to feel that each part of your body is losing sensation. What you should do is to try to remove any tension you feel in your body's any part totally. Don't suppress the thoughts if they occur; merely continue to direct your attention to the systematic relaxation of the different parts of the body in the way already mentioned. If you have managed to carry out these instruction in the way described, with awareness (that is important) you will surely feel that you have attained a wounderful relaxed state, physically and mentally. When you have finished the practice, gently move and clutch your hands, move your feet and slowly open your eyes.

If you are able to do this daily even for five minutes you would find a sea-change in your life. Particularly those people who remain under tension and charged state due to stress of the modern life which makes them lose hair profusely would find their hair regaining the lost shine and vitality. This is a very important asana and a virtual boon in the modern life. It relaxes the whole physiological and psychological system of the entire body and makes it acquire a beatific countenance.

❑

13

Your Diet in Hair Care

It is platitudinous to stress that a nutritious diet is essential for our growth and hence for the growth of hair also. But since physiologically hair is the least important of all human organs it gets minimum nutrition from the blood that which is left over after the vital organs have consumed the nutrition. But since it is a very much part of our body, it displays the first signs of nutritional deficiency when the problem disturbs the body. It is that signal which tells you that all is not well with your body. Normally it is believed that baldness is a hereditary disease but it can be checked if you can care well for your hair. After all no two human beings are identical so they can't have identical deficiencies. In most of the cases, in fact, it is the wrong practice adopted by your ancestors and maintained by you that you suffer most of the so-called hereditary diseases take for example the case of diabetes. It has been found that traditionally the Hindus have it more because their forefathers had put various restrictions in diets owing to their religious misconceptions. If you can have your logical sense involved in what and when and how you eat, certainly you can break this vicious hereditary cycle.

The same is true with hair. As already explained hair is

an extension of your skin and is composed of cells that have risen from generative cells deeper within the body-cells which get formed six to eight weeks earlier. Since hair is made up of protein called Keratin, hair needs protein for its growth and well- being. Now there are some super protein food items which the latest researches have found to be extremely good for hair.

Iodine Rich Items : It has been found that those who consume iodine rich diet have their hair strong and firm. Generally the people, particularly the ladies, living on the coastal regions have their hair invariably lush in thick; the credit for it is given to their fish-diet. There are certain varieties of fish like Rohu which have high content of iodine. Traditionally eating Jamun (plum) has also been found good for hair because of the rich content of iodine. For the same reason brinjal-diet is also found to be encouraging hair growth.

Eggs : These contain the largest amino acid, 'Methionine' than any other complete vitamin. Additionally eggs contain large quantities of vitamin A, B, D and E. Also they are rich in Sulphur content.

Milk : Milk is traditionally believed to be encouraging hair growth. There is an interesting poem by the famous medical Hindi poet Surdas in which Lord Krishna, in his childhood asks his mother as to why his 'Choti' (locks of hair) is not growing and the answer he receives is that he should drink more milk. Remember that milk is not meant for kids but for everyone. Many people claim that it is only humans that consume milk other than their mother's milk. They argue that since no other species requires milk, why must only humans consume it. But their argument is fallacious. For, the cow's milk (or for that matter even buffalo's milk) is a complete protein with built-in extra vitamins and minerals that spell lovely hair. Having a glass of milk when you retire is highly recommended if you want to retain your 'crowning glory'. Other milk products, particularly 'paneer' is very good for hair as well.

Yoghurt (Dahi or Curds) : This oldest health food has been treated as a solid tonic for hair not only through internal consumption but also through external application. Since it

110

contains lactic acid in adequate quantity—as is clear from a little sour taste—with all the nutrients and proteins in their most easily digestion form, it is easily assimilated by people of all categories. Moreover the curds are even otherwise a very liberal source of Vitamin B complex along with the bacteria which are extremely helpful in digestion. Hence curds are a must for those who wish to retain lush hair on their scalps. It is also treated as ideal to kill adverse effect of the antibiotic treatment. As the name suggests this treatment is inherently against life. The moment this treatment starts the body, in general, receives a negative effect. The activity of the living cells is drastically curtailed since the theory believes that the best way to get rid of any affliction is by starving it; that is by lessening all the vitalising activities of the body. But curds have those bacterial that reset the vitalisation function of the body. So those who have been or being treated by this kind of treatment must have at least hundred grams of curds everyday. Especially the pregnant ladies can fight against their inevitable hair-loss by consuming more and more of curds. It contains the bacteria which are very good for skin and hair.

Soyabean : A rich source of digestible protein, it is also good for hair. But make sure you have them in proper way, otherwise undigested soyabean might disturb the acid mantle of your scalp.

Sunflower Seeds : Also a good source of complete protein, high in poly-unsaturated fatty acids, rich in vitamins and minerals, these seeds in any form are good for hair.

Various Vitamins : A normal healthy body through the food it consumes, produces enough vitamins to meet its requirement. Then it is not needed to have vitamin tablets or other mineral supplement. Vitamins 'A', 'D', 'E' and 'K' can cause liver damage if taken in excess. The vitamins of B complex group are easily soluble in water and the body will take up only what it requires. And we know very well that vitamin 'B' is essential for healthy skin and has been considered the 'nerves' food. This also helps considerably in lessening and, even eliminating in some cases, like premenstrual tension. Since yeast contains much of it, having enough of yeast everyday is highly recommended for those who have hair problems. But preferably it should be in as natural a form as is edible. The composition of a yeast cell is very similar to the composition of the cells that make up the human body.

What You Should Avoid

It is a common knowledge that what is not good for one organ cannot be good of any other organ of a body. Hence the enemy of your body is also the enemy of your hair. So when we make our diet chart we must give margin to the toxins and poisons inevitably passing into our body with highly nutrient items. Of course we don't eat poison as such but you can't avoid slush from rain. It means that they have some of those items brought into the body which it can't digest. These have to be removed from the body. And the organs through which they are excreted include kidney, bowel, liver, lungs and sweat glands or the skin. It is when the body's scavenging system loses its efficiency that these toxins start accumulating over various parts of our body, particularly the skin, causing various diseases, symptoms. These symptoms cast the shadows of their appearance by manifesting themselves in different forms like boils, blisters or dandruff. In this sense we can class almost all of the snack items as enemies of hair like. Wafers/chips (particularly of potato) cakes, pastries, unrefined rice, maida, soft-white bread and other foods with high level of carbohydrates. All the fizzy drinks like Coke, Pepsi etc. have such toxic ingredients as are likely to damage our hair.

Hair grows best when you live close to nature. Air-conditioned living and tinned-food eating life can't expect as lustrous growth of hair as had made the poets think of the similes like-thick dense, rain-laden clouds.

❏ ❏